Johne's Disease

Guest Editor

MICHAEL T. COLLINS, DVM, PhD

VETERINARY CLINICS OF NORTH AMERICA: FOOD ANIMAL PRACTICE

www.vetfood.theclinics.com

Consulting Editor
ROBERT A. SMITH, DVM, MS

November 2011 • Volume 27 • Number 3

SAUNDERS an imprint of ELSEVIER, Inc.

W.B. SAUNDERS COMPANY
A Division of Elsevier Inc.

1600 John F. Kennedy Boulevard • Suite 1800 • Philadelphia, PA 19103-2899

http://www.vetfood.theclinics.com

VETERINARY CLINICS OF NORTH AMERICA: FOOD ANIMAL PRACTICE Volume 27, Number 3
November 2011 ISSN 0749-0720, ISBN-13: 978-1-4557-1041-6

Editor: John Vassallo; j.vassallo@elsevier.com
Developmental Editor: Teia Stone

Veterinary Clinics of North America: Food Animal Practice (ISSN 0749-0720) is published in March, July, and November by Elsevier Inc., 360 Park Avenue South, New York, NY 10010-1710. Subscription prices are $199.00 per year (domestic individuals), $278.00 per year (domestic institutions), $93.00 per year (domestic students/ residents), $225.00 per year (Canadian individuals), $363.00 per year (Canadian institutions), $284.00 per year (international individuals), $363.00 per year (international institutions), and $142.00 per year (international and Canadian students/ residents). To receive student/resident rate, orders must be accompanied by name of affiliated institution, date of term, and the signature of program/residency coordinator on institution letterhead. *Clinics* subscription prices. All prices are subject to change without notice. **POSTMASTER:** Send address changes to *Veterinary Clinics of North America: Food Animal Practice*, Elsevier Health Sciences Division, Subscription Customer Service, 3251 Riverport Lane, Maryland Heights, MO 63043. Customer Service (orders, claims, online, change of address): Elsevier Health Sciences Division, Subscription Customer Service, 3251 Riverport Lane, Maryland Heights, MO 63043. Tel: 1-800-654-2452 (U.S. and Canada); 314-447-8871 (ouside U.S. and Canada). Fax: 314-447-8029. E-mail: journalscustomerservice-usa@elsevier.com (for print support); journalsonlinesupport-usa@elsevier.com (for online support).

Reprints. For copies of 100 or more, of articles in this publication, please contact the Commercial Reprints Department, Elsevier Inc., 360 Park Avenue South, New York, NY 10010-1710. Tel.: 212-633-3812; Fax: 212-462-1935; E-mail: reprints@elsevier.com.

Veterinary Clinics of North America: Food Animal Practice is covered in *Current Contents/Agriculture, Biology and Environmental Sciences, MEDLINE/PubMed (Index Medicus),* and *Excerpta Medica.*

Printed and bound by CPI Group (UK) Ltd, Croydon, CR0 4YY

Transferred to Digital Print 2011

Contributors

CONSULTING EDITOR

ROBERT A. SMITH, DVM, MS
Diplomate, American Board of Veterinary Practitioners; Veterinary Research and Consulting Services, LLC, Greeley, Colorado

GUEST EDITOR

MICHAEL T. COLLINS, DVM, PhD
Diplomate, American College of Veterinary Internal Medicine; Professor of Microbiology, Department of Pathobiological Sciences, School of Veterinary Medicine, University of Wisconsin, Madison, Wisconsin

AUTHORS

MICHAEL A. CARTER, DVM, MPH
Assistant Director, Ruminant Health Programs, National Center for Animal Health Programs, Veterinary Services, Animal and Plant Health Inspection Service, US Department of Agriculture, Riverdale, Maryland

MICHAEL T. COLLINS, DVM, PhD
Diplomate, American College of Veterinary Internal Medicine; Professor of Microbiology, Department of Pathobiological Sciences, School of Veterinary Medicine, University of Wisconsin, Madison, Wisconsin

MARIE-EVE FECTEAU, DVM
Diplomate, American College of Veterinary Internal Medicine; Assistant Professor of Food Animal Medicine and Surgery, Department of Clinical Studies–New Bolton Center, School of Veterinary Medicine, University of Pennsylvania, Kennett Square, Pennsylvania

FRANKLYN GARRY, DVM, MS
Diplomate, American College of Veterinary Internal Medicine; Professor, Department of Clinical Sciences, Integrated Livestock Management, Colorado State University, Fort Collins, Colorado

DAVID KENNEDY, BVSc, MVS, MACVSc
AusVet Animal Health Services Pty Ltd, Orange, New South Wales, Australia

BRIAN W. KIRKPATRICK, MS, PhD
Professor of Animal Sciences and Dairy Science, Departments of Animal Sciences and Dairy Science, University of Wisconsin-Madison, Madison, Wisconsin

JASON E. LOMBARD, DVM, MS
Dairy Specialist/Veterinary Epidemiologist, National Animal Health Monitoring System (NAHMS), United States Department of Agriculture, Animal Plant Health Inspection Service, Veterinary Services, Centers for Epidemiology and Animal Health, Fort Collins, Colorado

ELIZABETH J.B. MANNING, MPH, MBA, DVM
Johne's Information Center, School of Veterinary Medicine, University of Wisconsin–Madison, Madison, Wisconsin

ELISABETH A. PATTON, DVM, PhD
Diplomate, American College of Veterinary Internal Medicine; Veterinary Program Manager, Wisconsin Department of Agriculture, Trade and Consumer Protection, Division of Animal Health, Madison, Wisconsin

SUELEE ROBBE-AUSTERMAN, DVM, MS, PhD
Head, Mycobacteria Brucella Section, Diagnostic Bacteriology Laboratory, National Veterinary Services Laboratories, United States Department of Agriculture, Animal Plant Health Inspection Service, Veterinary Services, Ames, Iowa

ALLEN J. ROUSSEL, DVM, MS
Diplomate, American College of Veterinary Internal Medicine; Diplomate, European College of Bovine Health Management; Professor, Department of Large Animal Clinical Sciences, Texas A&M University, College Station, Texas

GEORGE E. SHOOK, MS, PhD
Emeritus Professor of Dairy Science, University of Wisconsin-Madison, Madison, Wisconsin

RAYMOND W. SWEENEY, VMD
Diplomate, American College of Veterinary Internal Medicine; Professor of Medicine, Chief, Section of Large Animal Internal Medicine, Department of Clinical Studies–New Bolton Center, School of Veterinary Medicine, University of Pennsylvania, Kennett Square, Pennsylvania

ROBERT H. WHITLOCK, DVM, PhD
Diplomate, American College of Veterinary Internal Medicine; Associate Professor of Large Animal Medicine, Department of Clinical Studies–New Bolton Center, School of Veterinary Medicine, University of Pennsylvania, Kennett Square, Pennsylvania

Contents

> Johne's disease is the clinical manifestation of *Mycobacterium avium* subsp. *paratuberculosis* (MAP) infection and has become widespread since it was first observed in the United States in the early 1900s. MAP is primarily spread through the fecal-oral route, and herds generally become infected by unknowingly purchasing infected animals. The economic losses from the disease are primarily due to decreased milk production, decreased weaning weights in nursing young stock, increased replacement costs, and decreased slaughter value.

> Paratuberculosis in ruminants is characterized by oral ingestion of *Mycobacterium avium* subsp. *paratuberculosis* (MAP), followed by a long incubation period during which time MAP is able to survive within the host's macrophages. Initially the infection is held in check by the host's cell-mediated immune response, but gradually the host loses control of the infection. The infection incites a granulomatous inflammatory response in intestinal tissue and mesenteric lymph nodes, resulting in protein-losing enteropathy, malabsorption, diarrhea, weight loss, and edema.

> There is no definitive cure for *Mycobacterium avium* subsp. *paratuberculosis* (MAP) infections, but several therapeutic agents may be used to alleviate clinical signs of Johne's disease (JD) in ruminants of significant value. Treatment has to be maintained for the life of the animal and treated animals usually continue to shed MAP. No drugs are approved for treatment of JD in the United States; any drug use is "extra-label." Isoniazid, rifampin, and clofazimine are most commonly used for treatment. Monensin, may aid in the prevention of infection in calves and to lower MAP fecal shedding in infected adult cattle.

Multiple studies indicate that host animal genetics play a role in susceptibility to *Mycobacterium avium* subsp. *paratuberculosis* (MAP) infection. However, due to differences in methods used to define MAP-infected animals and controls and differences in methods of genetic analysis, there is as yet no clear consensus on the genes or markers to reliably define the MAP infection susceptibility of any animal species. Meta-analysis of combined studies and larger studies will help resolve the situation in the coming years.

One vaccine, Mycopar, is licensed for use in US cattle. The vaccine reduces clinical disease and fecal shedding of *Mycobacterium avium* subsp. *paratuberculosis* (MAP). The vaccine is indicated for use in herds with a high MAP infection prevalence or herds with limited resources for implementing paratuberculosis control measures. In heavily infected herds, a combination of vaccination and disease control measures can help protect susceptible young stock while reducing environmental burdens and limiting MAP transmission. There are regulatory restrictions on use of the vaccine and practitioners must consult their state veterinarian for guidance. Vaccines used in other countries have been widely adopted in Johne's disease control programs for small ruminants.

There is a wide array of accurate and affordable diagnostic tests for Johne's disease. The challenge is to be clear on the purpose for testing and then use the diagnostic test appropriate to that purpose for the specific animal species or type of business.

As with any susceptible livestock species, the key to control of paratuberculosis in beef cattle is to reduce exposure of the susceptible calves to *Mycobacterium avium* subsp. *paratuberculosis* (MAP)–contaminated feces. Because beef calves remain with mature, potentially shedding cattle until weaning, control strategies are aimed at providing an environment with the least possible fecal burden and removing MAP shedders as soon as possible. Testing and culling or separation may be more important in beef cattle than in dairy cattle. Seedstock owners have greater potential for economic loss from paratuberculosis, making control program more financially attractive to them than to commercial beef cattle producers.

> Control of Johne's disease in dairy herds involves 3 basic steps: prevent exposure of calves to *Mycobacterium avium* subsp. *paratuberculosis* (MAP), identify and eliminate MAP-infected cows from the herd, and prevent entry of MAP-infected animals into the herd. Tailoring JD control programs to each specific dairy requires education of the producer and a full understanding of his/her goals, objectives, and resources.

> The clinical presentation of paratuberculosis in small ruminants is unthriftiness (poor body condition); severe diarrhea is not a common clinical sign. In the USA, goats are primarily infected with bovine strains of paratuberculosis and sheep are primarily infected with ovine strains. Because ovine strains cannot be easily cultured, confirmation of a diagnosis is best done by polymerase chain reaction on tissue or fecal samples. Control programs must be tailored to the business objectives of the herd/flock owner and primarily involved changes in herd management, with diagnostic testing used strategically.

> All ruminant species, exotic or domestic, captive or free-ranging, are susceptible to disease and death due to *Mycobacterium avium* subsp. *paratuberculosis* (MAP) infection. Young ruminants are the most prone to infection through fecal-oral transmission. Fatal Johne's disease cases have occurred in numerous zoologic hoofstock collections and thus MAP infection is of concern for an industry focused on conserving rare individual animals and their genetics. Diagnosis is best based on MAP detection by PCR or culture in non-domestic species. True nonruminant wildlife reservoirs (ie, a population capable of sustaining the infection independently of reinfection from the initial source and transmitting the pathogen to other species) are rare.

> Both ante mortem and post mortem contamination of foods of animal origin commonly occurs. Food manufacturing practices fail to reliably kill *Mycobacterium avium* subsp. *paratuberculosis* (MAP) due to its innate resistance to heat and other physical factors. While medical science does not agree on the human health consequences of MAP exposure, this potentially zoonotic pathogen is found in a significant proportion of people with a disease bearing marked similarity to

Johne's disease (ie, Crohn's disease). Control of MAP infections in farm animals to mitigate the risk of human exposure is one additional reason for on-farm measures to control Johne's disease.

Paratuberculosis control in the United States has a long history, but only since 2002 has the US Department of Agriculture (USDA) had a formal control program in place. Modeled after work by the United States Animal Health Association (USAHA), the program continues to be a voluntary effort by states and producers. Education on paratuberculosis continues to be heavily emphasized by states.

Johne's disease has spread with livestock movements across the globe during the past century. International interest and collaboration in research and disease control have increased in the past 20 years. Control within infected herds and flocks has traditionally focused on reducing the impacts on animal welfare and productivity. Endemically infected regions are also moving to reduce contamination of the farm environment and of farm products. Several countries have been working to safeguard apparently free livestock populations and regions.

FORTHCOMING ISSUES

March 2012

Evidence-Based Veterinary Medicine for the Bovine Veterinarian
Sébastien Buczinski, Dr Vét and Jean-Michel Vandeweerd, DVM, MS, MRCVS, *Guest Editors*

July 2012

Mastitis
Pamela L. Ruegg, DVM, MPVM, *Guest Editor*

November 2012

Diagnostic Pathology
Vickie L. Cooper, DVM, MS, PhD, *Guest Editor*

RECENT ISSUES

July 2011

Ruminant Toxicology
Gary D. Osweiler, DVM, MS, PhD, *Guest Editor*

March 2011

Therapeutics and Control of Sheep and Goat Diseases
George C. Fthenakis, DVM, MSc, PhD, and Paula I. Menzies, DVM, MPVM, *Guest Editors*

November 2010

Production Animal Ophthalmology
David L. Williams, MA, VetMB, PhD, CertVOphthal, FRCVS, *Guest Editor*

RELATED INTEREST

Veterinary Clinics of North America: Equine Practice
April 2011 (Vol. 27, No. 1)
Endocrine Diseases
Ramiro E. Toribio, DVM, MS, PhD, *Guest Editor*

THE CLINICS ARE NOW AVAILABLE ONLINE!

Access your subscription at:
www.theclinics.com

Preface

Johne's Disease

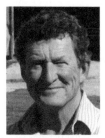

Michael T. Collins, DVM, PhD
Guest Editor

From the late 1800s to 1996, Johne's disease (paratuberculosis) spread among domesticated ruminants globally, emerging as one of the more common and costly ruminant infectious diseases, and prompting publication of the July 1996 issue of *Veterinary Clinics of North America: Food Animal Practice* devoted to Johne's disease guest edited under the guidance of Dr Ray Sweeney.[1] Since then, there has been a surge in research and development of national Johne's disease control programs around the world. The Johne's Disease Integrated Program in the United States invested over $8 million in applied and basic research on the etiology, *Mycobacterium avium* subsp. *paratuberculosis*.[2] In Europe, a multinational European Union program named ParaTBTools stimulated research similar in size and scope.[3] The products of these research programs are evident among the 2305 scientific publications from 1,465 institutions and 5149 authors between 1995 and 2009.[4]

This issue of *Veterinary Clinics of North America: Food Animal Practice* captures this wealth of new knowledge about Johne's disease and translates it into practical terms for veterinary practitioners. Authors of the enclosed articles are internationally recognized experts who work with practitioners and producers on a daily basis, giving them insights on Johne's disease only gained by years of experience and considerable trial and error. This issue provides a basic understanding of Johne's disease epidemiology and pathobiology, practical methods for Johne's disease control on farms, early information on genetic resistance, a description of national and international control efforts, and a glimpse into the future as to whether MAP is a human health issue: a zoonotic pathogen

Vet Clin Food Anim 27 (2011) xi–xii
doi:10.1016/j.cvfa.2011.08.001
0749-0720/11/$ – see front matter © 2011 Elsevier Inc. All rights reserved.

contaminating foods of animal-origin. I gratefully acknowledge the expertise and collegiality of my colleagues authoring this issue.

Michael T. Collins, DVM, PhD
Department of Pathobiological Sciences
School of Veterinary Medicine
University of Wisconsin
2015 Linden Drive
Madison, WI 53706, USA

E-mail address:
mcollin5@wisc.edu

REFERENCES

1. Sweeney RW, editor. Paratuberculosis (Johne's Disease). Vet Clin North Am Food Anim Pract 1996;12(2).
2. JDIP. http://www.jdip.org/. Accessed August 18, 2011.
3. ParaTBtools. http://www.vigilanciasanitaria.es/paratbtools/index.php. Accessed August 18, 2011.
4. Kaefska M, Hruska K. Analysis of publications on paratuberculosis from 1995 to 2009 with emphasis on the period from 2005 to 2009. Vet Med 2010;55:43–54.

Epidemiology and Economics of Paratuberculosis

Jason E. Lombard, DVM, MS

KEYWORDS

• Johne's • Paratuberculosis • Epidemiology • Prevalence
• Economics

Paratuberculosis, or Johne's disease (JD), is caused by the bacterium *Mycobacterium avium* subsp. *paratuberculosis* (MAP). Although JD is frequently used in discussing MAP infections, the use of JD technically should be restricted to the clinical manifestation of MAP infection; the preclinical stage being called paratuberculosis. The first reported occurrence of JD, which was initially thought to be an intestinal form of tuberculosis, was in the early 1800s in Germany and was later described by Drs Johne and Frothingham.[1] In the United States, the first reported case of JD appeared in Pennsylvania in 1908.[2] The disease has since been observed in cattle, other ruminants, and various other domestic and wild animals worldwide.[3] Most of the research on MAP infection has focused on cattle, dairy cattle in particular.

Calves and other ruminants less than 6 months of age are generally considered to be at the greatest risk of becoming infected with MAP. Neonates are likely the most susceptible due to increased permeability of the intestines in the first 24 hours of life.[4,5] Although there are data to support infection of adult cattle with MAP,[6] calfhood infection is far more important in most herd situations. The average incubation period of MAP infection in dairy cattle has been estimated at 5 years,[7] with the incubation period being inversely related to the MAP dose—that is, the more MAP consumed, the shorter time period before displaying clinical signs. Some infected cattle may not show clinical signs within their productive lifetime.[8] One of the difficulties in controlling MAP infection is that animals frequently shed MAP in feces prior to showing any clinical signs, thus insidiously contributing to spread of the infection.

A report from the 1920s suggested that MAP infection was present at low levels in the US cattle population.[9] The report warned that the problem should be dealt with before it became endemic like tuberculosis and brucellosis were at the time. The interesting aspect of the history of MAP infection in the United States is that our

The author has nothing to disclose.
National Animal Health Monitoring System (NAHMS), United States Department of Agriculture, Animal Plant Health Inspection Service, Veterinary Services, Centers for Epidemiology and Animal Health, 2150 Centre Avenue, Building B-2E7, Fort Collins, CO 80526-8117, USA
E-mail address: Jason.E.Lombard@aphis.usda.gov

Vet Clin Food Anim 27 (2011) 525–535
doi:10.1016/j.cvfa.2011.07.012
0749-0720/11/$ – see front matter © 2011 Elsevier Inc. All rights reserved.

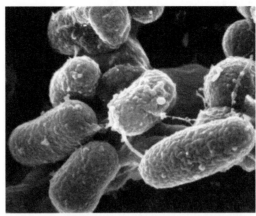

Fig. 1. Scanning electron micrograph of *Mycobacterium avium* subsp. *paratuberculosis*, ×50,000 magnification. (*Courtesy of* Michael T. Collins, DVM, PhD, Madison, WI.)

predecessors not only predicted the disease would continue to spread but also recommended diagnostic tests and control strategies that remain the basis of current programs.[10] Unfortunately, despite the early warnings and availability of diagnostic tools, the infection has continued to spread. The tools currently available (diagnostic tests and control programs) will be discussed in depth in other articles in this issue.

MAP: CHARACTERISTICS, ENVIRONMENTAL PERSISTENCE, AND HEAT RESISTANCE

MAP is a gram-positive, acid-fast organism that has a rough, thick, and waxy cell wall (**Fig. 1**). All *Mycobacterium* species other than MAP produce the iron-chelating agent mycobactin.[1] Since iron is required for replication, MAP is considered an obligate parasite of mammalian cells where iron is readily available to the organism and mycobactin is not needed.[11] MAP preferentially infects macrophages upon entry into the host and thus is considered a facultative intracellular pathogen.[12,13]

The tenacious, protective cell wall and propensity to form large clumps of cells allows MAP to withstand a variety of harsh conditions and survive for longer than 1 year in the environment.[14] A study of naturally infected sheep feces found that direct sunlight and UV radiation had the greatest negative impact on MAP survival. Shade, even in the form of grass, increased MAP survival time.[15]

In addition to withstanding a variety of environmental conditions, the organism is resistant to heat and has been shown to survive high-temperature, short-time pasteurization (72°C for 15 seconds) if present in sufficient numbers in raw milk.[16] Batch pasteurization of colostrum at 60°C (140°F) for 60 minutes is sufficient to eliminate MAP under most conditions.[17] In a controlled study, viable MAP was not detected in MAP-spiked waste milk samples after 30 minuites at 65.6°C.[18]

MAP PREVALENCE

Prevalence, an estimate of the number of infected animals in a population at a given time, is determined via testing of a sufficient number of animals to produce an estimate with the desired degree of precision. Prevalence can be reported as apparent (test) prevalence where the estimate is the number of animals that test positive divided by the total number of animals tested. Alternatively, true prevalence can be calculated by adjusting the apparent prevalence based on the accuracy of the test used. For example, if a test is used that detects 50% of MAP-infected animals (test sensitivity = 50%) and all animals that test positive are truly infected (test specificity = 100%), then the true prevalence would be twice the apparent prevalence. More complex methods exist for estimating true prevalence from test prevalence data by including the impact of test specificity as well as variability associated with test characteristics under various use conditions. Estimates of MAP prevalence are commonly reported, but differences in sampling design and diagnostic strategies make direct comparison of the studies difficult.[19] Fecal culture and enzyme-linked immunosorbent assay (ELISA) for antibodies in serum or milk have been the most common diagnostic methods used determining MAP infection prevalence.

There is evidence that the prevalence of MAP infection has increased since first detected in the United States in the early 1900s. And although there are limited data to support the notion that that animal-level prevalence has increased, it is well accepted that the herd-level prevalence of MAP-infected dairy herds has increased. Reasons for the increase in herd-level prevalence include the ongoing consolidation of the dairy industry and continued purchasing of subclinically MAP-infected animals by previously uninfected herds. Both of these reasons are supported from data collected during the NAHMS Dairy 2007 study, where herd-level prevalence increased as herd size increased and a higher percentage of MAP-infected herds purchased dairy replacements compared with uninfected herds.[20]

Animal-Level Prevalence

Many studies have been conducted in the United States as well as in other countries to estimate animal-level prevalence in cattle. Few estimates for prevalence of MAP infection in small ruminants in the United States have been reported. In general, estimates have been higher for dairy cattle than for beef cattle and for estimates of cattle going through a market (sale barn) or at slaughter compared with on-farm testing. The dairy cow-level prevalence of MAP infection in the United States has ranged from 1% to 20%, with the average being 5% to 10%. Specific country-level estimates for dairy cattle ranged from 1.2% in Belgium[21] to 8.8% in Denmark.[22] The most recent estimate for the United States was 2.5% but the study was conducted in 1996.[23] In beef cattle, the prevalence is generally less than 5% with very few countries reporting.

Herd-Level Prevalence

The herd-level prevalence of MAP infection for dairy operations is much higher than for beef operations in the United States and other countries. The NAHMS Dairy 2007 study of US herds in the top 17 dairy states estimated that more than 68% of US dairy herds are MAP infected based on testing of composite fecal samples.[24] Other studies focused on dairy herds in specific states have reported similar findings. Much lower herd-level prevalence estimates have been reported in beef cattle herds. The NAHMS Beef '97 study detected MAP infection in 7.9% of herds[25]; however, that study was designed only to detect MAP in herds with at least 10% of animals infected. Thus, the herd-level prevalence of MAP in beef herds is likely higher than 7.9% but is likely much lower than the herd-level prevalence for dairy herds.

Within-Herd Prevalence

Precise estimation of the within-herd prevalence of MAP infection in commercial dairy and beef cow-calf herds is generally not recommended primarily because of the cost involved in testing a sufficient number of cattle to obtain an accurate estimate.[26] Results of studies estimating within-herd prevalence in dairy operations have been variable and ranged from 0% to 70%.[27–30] Although high-prevalence herds exist, the majority of infected herds have low to moderate MAP infection prevalence. For example, the NAHMS Dairy 2002 study reported within-herd seroprevalence levels from 0% to 27.3% with a mean of 5.5% for the 106 operations evaluated.[30] Estimates of within-herd prevalence for beef operations are rare. Estimates from 25 herds enrolled in the National Johne's Disease Demonstration Herd Project ranged from 0 to 20% (Chuck Fossler, DVM, PhD, Fort Collins, CO, personal communication, November 2010).

Higher within-herd prevalence tends to be associated with MAP shedding in feces at a younger age. Higher prevalence levels are likely associated with higher MAP exposure, which results in relatively shorter incubation periods and clinical signs in younger animals compared to herds with lower within-herd prevalence. Additionally, as the prevalence increases, more JD cases will likely be observed. The number of clinical cases observed over a specific time period is often used as a proxy for the within-herd prevalence. However, this estimate can be misleading if the animals with JD were recently purchased.

TRANSMISSION
Transmission—Within Herd

Three routes of infection have been proposed: fecal-oral, congenital, and through mammary secretions. Calves less than 6 months of age are generally considered to be at the greatest risk of becoming MAP infected with neonates likely being the most susceptible due to increased permeability of the intestines in the first 24 hours of life.[4,5]

The primary route of MAP transmission in all species is thought to be fecal-oral[31,32] with bacteria-laden manure being the primary source of infection.[33] The presence of lesions within the intestine and the large numbers of MAP bacteria shed in the feces support fecal contamination/ingestion as the primary source of new infections within a herd. Fecal contamination of the teats/udder or calving environment is thought to be the primary risk factor for neonatal infection.[19] A "super-shedder" is an MAP-infected cow that sheds 100 to 1000 times more MAP than a typical "heavy shedder." These cows, if present in a herd, likely represent the greatest source of MAP contamination of the environment and primary source of new infections.[6]

MAP has been isolated from milk and colostrum of cows during subclinical and clinical stages of infection. In a study of subclinically infected cows, shedding of MAP in colostrum (22.2% of cows) was 3 times greater than in milk (8.3%), indicating the importance of colostrum as a mode of transmission.[34] Thirty-five percent of cows with advanced clinical disease were also found to have MAP in their milk.[35] Additionally, colostrum and milk may become contaminated during milking if the teats are not properly cleaned and disinfected prior to harvest. The feeding of pooled colostrum and/or milk increases risk of MAP transmission since there is a greater chance that at least one cow in the pool is shedding MAP, and more calves are exposed than if single-source colostrum or milk was fed to each calf.

Transplacental transmission has also been documented in cows clinically and subclinically MAP infected. Although the mechanism of fetal/transplacental infection is not currently known, theories include uterine contamination of the embryo and hematogenous or lymphatic spread to the developing embryo/fetus. Approximately 17% of cows that were subclinically MAP infected delivered calves that were tissue culture positive for MAP.[36] Another study evaluating subclinically and clinically infected cows found 26.4% of calves to be culture positive.[37] A meta-analysis conducted by Whittington and Windsor[38] estimated that about 9% of fetuses from subclinically infected cows and 39% of fetuses from clinically affected cows were MAP infected.

Other potential modes of transmission include venereal,[39,40] via rectal examination,[41] and during embryo transfer procedures.[42] However, a limited study evaluating low to moderate MAP shedders found no evidence that oocytes or embryos harbor the bacteria when processed according to current embryo transfer recommendations.[43]

While fecal-oral transmission is widely regarded as the primary means of MAP transmission, it is possible that other routes may play a role. An editorial in *The Veterinary Journal* raised questions about the current knowledge of the transmission of MAP.[44] The authors present the analogy of *Mycobacterium bovis*, the causative agent of bovine tuberculosis, and the long-held belief that the bacterium was transmitted via the fecal-oral route. Eventually, it was documented that transmission occurred via the aerosol route. The authors propose that all potential routes of MAP transmission be explored rather than just fecal-oral. MAP has also been detected in dust samples in housing facilities of an infected herd suggesting that the organism can become airborne and spread via aerosols.[45] Although the majority of evidence supports the traditional fecal-oral route as the important infection transmission route, a study reported finding the organism only in tracheobronchial lymph nodes supporting the occurrence of aerosol transmission.[46]

Specific risk factors for within-herd transmission are difficult to identify since most studies are cross-sectional and management practices to limit transmission often have already been implemented by owners of MAP-infected animals at the time of a study, making those practices appear to increase transmission when, in fact, they decrease transmission. For an individual herd, the various risks of MAP transmission must be evaluated and addressed in decreasing order of importance. Implementations of practices to limit transmission are generally herd-specific (ie, there is not a single protocol for decreasing within-herd MAP transmission for all herds).

The calving area and calf rearing practices should be the major focus of any control program. Implementation of recommended manage practices to control MAP has increased in the United States, but there is still room for improvement. For example, almost one-third of herds of more than 500 dairy cows allowed test-positive cows in the calving area. Separating the calf from the dam has been promoted to reduce transmission and the percentage of dairy herds that separate calves immediately has increased from 28.0% of herds in 1991 to 55.9% in 2007. Colostrum from test-positive dams was reportedly fed to calves on almost 5% of US dairy herds. Pooling of colostrum was reported by 21% of herds but was a more common practice in herds of 500 cows or more, so a large percentage of dairy calves in the United States are being fed pooled colostrum. Colostrum and milk was routinely pasteurized on only 0.8% and 4.2% of dairy herds, respectively.[47] Implementation of the above-recommended management practices along with attention to general hygiene are necessary for reducing within-herd transmission of MAP. Specific management practices for controlling MAP infection are presented in other articles in this issue.

Transmission—Between Herds

The most likely source of MAP introduction into a previously uninfected herd is from the purchase of infected cattle.[41] Other potential sources, although considered negligible compared to introduction of an infected animal, include manure movement between farms, purchase of colostrum or milk, and sharing of pastures or water sources. The risk of a herd becoming infected from wild animals appears to be minimal, and the more likely scenario is a potential spillover of infection in cattle or small ruminants to nearby wild animals. Off-site heifer raising presents another potential route of between-herd transmission. A study of waste milk delivered and fed to calves at 4 calf ranches found viable MAP present in the milk. Although MAP was present at low levels, one milk sample contained viable MAP even after on-farm pasteurization.[48]

Results from the NAHMS Dairy 2007 study are consistent with the claim that disease introduction occurs primarily through new herd additions. A higher percentage of dairy herds that brought in new additions in 2006 were MAP infected compared with uninfected herds.[20] Additionally, testing of incoming dairy cattle for MAP infection was performed by only 10% of US dairy herds over the time period 1996–2007.

For beef herds, the purchase of subclinically infected breeding bulls appears to be a major risk based on anecdotal reports. Since most beef operations raise their own replacement heifers and add new genetics through the purchase of bulls, it makes sense that purchasing bulls is the largest MAP infection risk. Additionally, the purchase of preweaned dairy calves to suckle beef cows that have lost their calf and the purchase of colostrum or raw milk from dairies can also be major risks for MAP introduction. The NAHMS Beef 2007–2008 study reported that only 2.1% of beef operations that had purchased cattle in the 3 years prior to the study tested herd additions for MAP infection. Introduction of new animals is a common practice among dairy and beef herds in the United States. Almost 4 of 10 dairy herds brought on new additions in 2006, while almost 7 of 10 beef herds brought on new additions in the 3 years prior to that study.[47,49]

ECONOMICS OF MAP INFECTION

When discussing the costs of MAP infection with producers, it is important to point out that typical "losses" are in the form of potential or unrealized revenue versus "out-of-pocket costs," and the goal of reducing the economic impact of MAP infection should be to decrease the amount of these "losses." When proposing a control program, which typically requires the producer to pay out-of-pocket costs, it is essential that the proposed plan does not cost the producer more than the decrease in potential revenue from MAP infected cattle. A Johne's Disease Cost Worksheet is available that gives a ballpark estimate of lost milk revenue, increased replacement costs, and the decreased revenue from the sale of infected cows.[50] Providing producers an estimate of what the disease is costing in terms of lost revenue is useful in determining how much to invest in a control program. However, it should be noted that efforts to control MAP transmission (eg, maintaining a clean calving area, removing calves immediately after birth, feeding single source colostrums) have collateral benefits; they also decrease transmission of other fecal-oral transmitted pathogens. The economic benefits of these practices in controlling other diseases have not been determined.

The economic impact of MAP infection in dairy herds with high prevalence is easy for producers to notice because they are seeing and selling cattle with JD. Herds with low prevalence may not have animals with clinical disease and may be unaware their herd is infected. The implementation of a control program specifically for MAP in low-prevalence herds is probably not cost effective unless they are in the business of selling breeding cattle. Herds that only occasionally observe an animal with JD require closer scrutiny to determine whether devotion of resources to control MAP is justifiable. However, if sufficient evidence arises in the future showing MAP causes human disease (ie, is a zoonotic pathogen), then the impetus for implementing MAP infection control measures could increase dramatically. The possible association of MAP and human disease is discussed in a later article in this issue.

Specific aspects of JD control programs for different animal species are covered in other chapters. It is important to point out that JD control programs do not necessarily incur costs to the producer. Education of producers about JD and recommendations to purchase animals from low MAP infection risk herds are fundamental parts of control programs that are essentially without cost. And, although MAP control programs, which should be part of any overall biosecurity program, are focused on a specific pathogen, they are generally effective against numerous disease-causing agents transmitted via the fecal-oral route.

Several studies have evaluated the economic impact of MAP infection in dairy herds but the results have been mixed. In general, MAP test-positive cows, even if not showing clinical signs of disease, produce less milk, are culled earlier in their productive life, and have lower salvage value compared with uninfected herd mates. Although reductions in first lactation milk production are inconsistently reported, decreased milk production in subsequent lactations is consistently found and can be from 4% to 20% lower than for test-negative herdmates.[51–57] The estimated monetary impact varies based on the how cattle are classified (eg, test-positive vs test-negative, by type of test used, and whether the cows have progressed to JD) and the milk and cattle prices used in the study.

Few studies have evaluated the impact of MAP infection on milk quality, reproduction, or the association with other common dairy cattle diseases and the results are not consistent. If MAP infection does impact these parameters, it is likely a small proportion of the overall economic costs.

MAP-infected cattle have been shown to be at twice the risk of being culled compared with uninfected herd mates,[58,59] even when producers were not aware of the animal's infection status.[56] Two studies have reported that test-positive cows average 30 to 54 kg (70–130 lb) less at removal than test-negative herd mates.[60,61] Infected cows were found to have a 30% decrease in market value, primarily because of lower salvage weight.[53]

One study reported that MAP infection in sheep caused significant economic loss due to deaths, with losses accounting on average for two-thirds of the total estimated financial loss associated with sheep deaths.[62] Studies on the economic impact of MAP infections in beef cattle and small ruminant herds are almost nonexistent. It is reasonable to assume that some of the same effects observed in dairy cattle also occur in beef cattle and small ruminants (eg, reduced milk production leading to lower weaning weights, loss of body condition with premature culling, and reduced salvage value). Although the impact of these potential effects has not been determined, beef producers who sell calves for feeding and slaughter would not incur a noticeable decrease in revenue associated with MAP infections in calves. However, MAP-infected cows may remain in the herd long enough to manifest JD, thus shortening the cow's productive life resulting in financial losses. The potential loss due to MAP infections for seedstock producers is much greater compared to commercial cow-calf operations since they could potentially lose their market for live animal sales.

SUMMARY

JD is the clinical manifestation of MAP infection and has become more widespread since it was first observed in the United States in the early 1900s. Most herds that become infected probably do so through the purchase of infected animals. This bacterial pathogen is primarily spread via the fecal-oral route or indirectly through fecal contamination of colostrum, milk, or feed. Economic losses are primarily due to lost or unrealized revenue (decreased milk and slaughter value) and not increased producers' expenditures. Implementation of a control program will likely, but not always, incur additional expenditures for the producer. The use of simple cost-of-disease calculations may help educate and identify those producers that need to address the problem. Every producer should have a biosecurity program that limits the chances for MAP introduction to and spread within their operation. Client education about JD is a necessary first step.

REFERENCES

1. Chiodini RJ, van Kruiningen HJ, Merkal RS. Ruminant paratuberculosis (Johne's disease): the current status and future prospects. Cornell Vet 1984;74(3):218–62.
2. Pearson L. A note on the occurrence in America of chronic bacterial dysentery of cattle. Am Vet Rev 1908;32:602–5.
3. Harris NB, Barletta RG. *Mycobacterium avium* subsp. *paratuberculosis* in Veterinary Medicine. Clin Microbiol Rev 2001;14(3):489–512.
4. Hagan WA. Age as a factor in susceptibility to Johne's disease. Cornell Vet 1938;28: 34–40.
5. Larsen AB, Merkal RS, Cutlip RC. Age of cattle as related to resistance to infection with *Mycobacterium paratuberculosis*. Am J Vet Res 1975;36(3):255–7.
6. Whitlock RH, Sweeney RW, Fyock TL, et al. MAP Super-Shedders: Another factor in the control of Johne's disease. In: Proceedings of the 8th International Colloquium on Paratuberculosis. Copenhagen, Denmark: 2005.
7. Jubb TF, Sergeant ES, Callinan AP, et al. Estimate of the sensitivity of an ELISA used to detect Johne's disease in Victorian dairy cattle herds. Aust Vet J 2004;82(9):569–73.
8. Whittington RJ, Sergeant ES. Progress towards understanding the spread, detection and control of *Mycobacterium avium* subsp *paratuberculosis* in animal populations. Aust Vet J 2001;79(4):267–78.
9. Beach BA, Hastings EG. Johne's disease: a cattle menace. UW-Madison, Agricultural Experiment Station Bulletin 343. 1922.
10. Moyle AI. Culture and cull procedure for control of paratuberculosis. J Am Vet Med Assoc 1975;166(7):689–90.
11. Lambrecht RS, Collins MT. Inability to detect mycobactin in mycobacteria-infected tissues suggests an alternative iron acquisition mechanism by mycobacteria in vivo. Microb Pathog 1993;14(3):229–38.
12. Thorel MF, Krichevsky M, Levy-Frebault VV. Numerical taxonomy of mycobactin-dependent mycobacteria, emended description of *Mycobacterium avium*, and description of *Mycobacterium avium* subsp. *avium* subsp. *nov.*, *Mycobacterium avium* subsp. *paratuberculosis* subsp. *nov.*, and *Mycobacterium avium* subsp. *silvaticum* subsp. *nov.* Int J Syst Bacteriol 1990;40(3):254–60.
13. Coussens PM. *Mycobacterium paratuberculosis* and the bovine immune system. Anim Health Res Rev 2001;2(2):141–61.
14. Larsen AB, Merkal RS, Vardaman TH. Survival time of *Mycobacterium paratuberculosis*. Am J Vet Res 1956;17(64):549–51.
15. Whittington RJ, Marshall DJ, Nicholls PJ, et al. Survival and dormancy of *Mycobacterium avium* subsp. *paratuberculosis* in the environment. Appl Environ Microbiol 2004;70(5):2989–3004.
16. Grant IR, Hitchings EI, McCartney A, et al. Effect of commercial-scale high-temperature, short-time pasteurization on the viability of *Mycobacterium paratuberculosis* in naturally infected cows' milk. Appl Environ Microbiol 2002;68(2):602–7.

17. Godden S, McMartin S, Feirtag J, et al. 2006. Heat-treatment of bovine colostrum. II: effects of heating duration on pathogen viability and immunoglobulin G. J Dairy Sci 89:3476–83.

18. Stabel JR. On-farm batch pasteurization destroys Mycobacterium paratuberculosis in waste milk. J Dairy Sci 2001;84(2):524–7.

19. NRC (National Research Council). Diagnosis and control of Johne's disease. Washington, DC: National Academies Press; 2003.

20. Lombard J, Capsel R, Wagner B, et al. Changes in management practices and herd-level prevalence of *Mycobacterium avium* subspecies *paratuberculosis* (MAP) infection on US Dairy operations. Proc Am Assoc Bov Pract 2008;41:242.

21. Boelaert F, Walravens K, Biront P, et al. Prevalence of paratuberculosis (Johne's disease) in the Belgian cattle population. Vet Microbiol 2000;77(3–4):269–81.

22. Jakobsen MB, Alban L, Nielsen SS. A cross-sectional study of paratuberculosis in 1155 Danish dairy cows. Prev Vet Med 2000;46(1):15–27.

23. USDA. Johne's disease on US dairy operations. Fort Collins (CO): USDA-APHIS-VS, CEAH, National Animal Health Monitoring System; 2008. N245.1097.

24. USDA. Johne's disease on US dairies, 1991–2007. Fort Collins (CO): USDA-APHIS-VS, CEAH, National Animal Health Monitoring System; 2008. N521.0408.

25. USDA. What do I need to know about Johne's disease in beef cattle? Fort Collins (CO): USDA-APHIS-VS, CEAH, National Animal Health Monitoring System; 1999. N309.899.

26. Collins MT, Gardner IA, Garry FB, et al. Consensus recommendations on diagnostic testing for the detection of paratuberculosis in cattle in the United States. J Am Vet Med Assoc 2006;229(12):1912–9.

27. Collins MT, Sockett DC, Goodger WJ, et al. Herd prevalence and geographic distribution of, and risk factors for, bovine paratuberculosis in Wisconsin. J Am Vet Med Assoc 1994;204(4):636–41.

28. Obasanjo IO, Grohn YT, Mohammed HO. Farm factors associated with the presence of *Mycobacterium paratuberculosis* infection in dairy herds on the New York State Paratuberculosis Control Program. Prev Vet Med 1997;32(3–4):243–51.

29. Hirst HL. Johne's disease on Colorado Dairies: Association of herd characteristics with seroprevlaence and behavior of an ELISA when cattle were resampled at two to twenty month intervals. Master's thesis. Colorado State University, Department of Clinical Sciences; 2001.

30. USDA. Johne's disease on US dairy operations, 2002. Fort Collins (CO): USDA-APHIS-VS, CEAH, National Animal Health Monitoring System; 2005. N427.0205.

31. Clarke CJ. The pathology and pathogenesis of paratuberculosis in ruminants and other species. J Comp Pathol 1997;116(3):217–61.

32. Stehman SM. Paratuberculosis in small ruminants, deer, and South American camelids. Vet Clin North Am Food Anim Pract 1996;12(2):441–55.

33. Larsen AB. Paratuberculosis: the status of our knowledge. J Am Vet Med Assoc 1972;161(11):1539–41.

34. Streeter RN, Hoffsis GF, Bech-Nielsen S, et al. Isolation of *Mycobacterium paratuberculosis* from colostrum and milk of subclinically infected cows. Am J Vet Res 1995;56(10):1322–4.

35. Taylor TK, Wilks CR, McQueen DS. Isolation of *Mycobacterium paratuberculosis* from the milk of a cow with Johne's disease. Vet Rec 1981;109(24):532–3.

36. Sweeney RW, Whitlock RH, Rosenberger AE. *Mycobacterium paratuberculosis* isolated from fetuses of infected cows not manifesting signs of the disease. Am J Vet Res 1992c;53(4):477–80.

37. Seitz SE, Heider LE, Heuston WD, et al. Bovine fetal infection with *Mycobacterium paratuberculosis*. J Am Vet Med Assoc 1989;194(10):1423–6.
38. Whittington RJ, Windsor PA. In utero infection of cattle with *Mycobacterium avium* subsp. *paratuberculosis:* a critical review and meta-analysis. Vet J 2009;179(1):60–9.
39. Larsen AB, Stalheim OH, Hughes DE, et al. *Mycobacterium paratuberculosis* in the semen and genital organs of a semen-donor bull. J Am Vet Med Assoc 1981;179(2): 169–71.
40. Eppleston J, Whittington RJ. Isolation of *Mycobacterium avium* subsp *paratuberculosis* from the semen of rams with clinical Johne's disease. Aust Vet J 2001;79(11): 776–7.
41. Sweeney RW. Transmission of paratuberculosis. Vet Clin North Am Food Anim Pract 1996;12(2):305–12.
42. Rohde RF, Shulaw WP. Isolation of *Mycobacterium paratuberculosis* from the uterine flush fluids of cows with clinical paratuberculosis. J Am Vet Med Assoc 1990;197(11): 1482–3.
43. Kruip TA, Muskens J, van Roermund HJ, et al. Lack of association of *Mycobacterium avium* subsp. *paratuberculosis* with oocytes and embryos from moderate shedders of the pathogen. Theriogenology 2003;59(7):1651–60.
44. Corner LA, Pfeiffer DU, Abbott KA. Unanswered questions about the transmission of *Mycobacterium avium* subspecies *paratuberculosis*. Vet J 2003;165(3):182–3.
45. Eisenberg SW, Nielen M, Santema W, et al. Detection of spatial and temporal spread of *Mycobacterium avium* subsp. *paratuberculosis* in the environment of a cattle farm through bio-aerosols. Vet Microbiol 2010;143(2–4):284–92. Epub 2009 Dec 3.
46. Pavlik I, Matlova L, Bartl J, et al. Parallel faecal and organ *Mycobacterium avium* subsp. *paratuberculosis* culture of different productivity types of cattle. Vet Microbiol 2000;77(3–4):309–24.
47. USDA. Biosecurity practices on US dairy operations, 1991–2007. Fort Collins (CO): USDA-APHIS-VS, CEAH, National Animal Health Monitoring System; 2010. N544.0510.
48. Ruzante JM, Gardner IA, Cullor JS, et al. Isolation of *Mycobacterium avium* subsp. *paratuberculosis* from waste milk delivered to California calf ranches. Foodborne Pathog Dis 2008;5(5):681–6.
49. USDA. Beef 2007–08. Part IV: Reference of beef cow-calf management practices in the United States, 2007–08. Fort Collins (CO): USDA-APHIS-VS, CEAH, National Animal Health Monitoring System; 2010. 523.0210.
50. NIAA. The cost of Johne's disease to dairy producers. National Institute for Animal Agriculture. Colorado (CO): Springs; 2009. 09-69224-00.
51. Buergelt CD, Duncan JR. Age and milk production data of cattle culled from a dairy herd with paratuberculosis. J Am Vet Med Assoc 1978;173(5 Pt 1):478–80.
52. Abbas B, Riemann HP, Hird DW. Diagnosis of Johne's disease (paratuberculosis) in Northern California cattle and a note on its economic significance. Calif Vet 1983;8: 20–4.
53. Benedictus G, Dijkhuizen AA, Stelwagen J. Economic losses due to paratuberculosis in dairy cattle. Vet Rec 1987;121(7):142–6.
54. Spangler E, Bech-Nielsen S, Heider LE. Diagnostic performance of two serologic tests and fecal culture for subclinical paratuberculosis, and associations with production. Prev Vet Med 1992;13:185–95.
55. Sweeney RW, Hutchinson LJ, Whitlock RH, et al. Effect of *Mycobacterium paratuberculosis* on milk production in dairy cattle. In: Proceedings of the 4th International Colloquium on Paratuberculosis. Cambridge (UK): Colloquium; 1995. p. 133–5.

56. Lombard JE, Garry FB, McCluskey BJ, et al. Risk of removal and effects on milk production associated with paratuberculosis status in dairy cows. J Am Vet Med Assoc 2005;227(12):1975–81.

57. Nordlund KV, Goodger WJ, Pelletier J, et al. Associations between subclinical paratuberculosis and milk production, milk components, and somatic cell counts in dairy herds. J Am Vet Med Assoc 1996;208(11):1872–6.

58. Wilson DJ, Rossiter C, Han HR, et al. Association of *Mycobacterium paratuberculosis* infection with reduced mastitis, but with decreased milk production and increased cull rate in clinically normal dairy cows. Am J Vet Res 1993;54(11):1851–7.

59. Goodell GM, Hirst HL, Garry FB, et al. Comparison of cull rates and milk production of clinically normal dairy cows grouped by ELISA *Mycobacterium avium paratuberculosis* serum antibody results. In: Proceedings International Society for Veterinary Epidemiology and Economics. Breckenridge, (CO): International Society for Veterinary Epidemiology and Economics; 2002. p. 897–9.

60. Whitlock RH, Hutchinson LJ, Merkal RS, et al. Prevalence and economic considerations of Johne's disease in Northeastern US. In: Proceedings, Annual Meeting of the United States Animal Health Association. Milwaukee (WI): United States Animal Health Association, 1985;98:484–90.

61. Johnson-Ifearulundu Y, Kaneene JB, Lloyd JW. Herd-level economic analysis of the impact of paratuberculosis on dairy herds. J Am Vet Med Assoc 1999;214(6):822–5.

62. Bush RD, Windsor PA, Toribio JA. Losses of adult sheep due to ovine Johne's disease in 12 infected flocks over a 3-year period. Aust Vet J 2006;84(7):246–53.

Pathogenesis of Paratuberculosis

Raymond W. Sweeney, VMD

KEYWORDS

- Johne's • Paratuberculosis • *Mycobacterium* • Ruminants
- Pathogenesis

TRANSMISSION

The etiologic agent of Johne's disease, *Mycobacterium avium* subsp. *paratuberculosis* (MAP), is most commonly transmitted by the fecal-oral route. Organisms shed in the feces of infected animals, usually adults, are ingested by susceptible, usually juvenile, animals. Due to its hearty nature, MAP has the capacity to survive for extended periods in the environment, so oral contact with contaminated surfaces such as maternity pen surfaces, bedding, dams' udders, or feeding utensils or consumption of feed or pasture contaminated with feces can result in ingestion of MAP. Furthermore, cows with paratuberculosis may also shed MAP directly in the milk or colostrum, so consumption of these products by susceptible calves can also result in infection.[1,2] Most new infections are thought to occur in young animals, often in the first few months, or even first days, of life. Additionally, in utero transmission of MAP from infected cow to fetus has been documented. In various studies, MAP has been recovered from up to 40% of fetuses from cows with clinical signs of paratuberculosis, from 18% of asymptomatic but "heavy shedding" cows (based on fecal MAP colony counts), and rarely from "light shedders."[3,4] It is presumed, but not known for sure, that prenatally (in utero) infected calves will have a similar clinical progression and pathogenesis as calves exposed postnatally by the oral route.

SUSCEPTIBILITY TO INFECTION

It has long been well established that resistance to infection with MAP increases with age.[5–9] Most experimental infection studies, as well as some field studies, have shown that between 4 months and 1 year of age, it becomes more difficult to infect calves, and that by 1 year of age susceptibility is probably similar to that of an adult. The mechanism for increased susceptibility of young calves has not been determined. It has been speculated that the "open gut" in the first 24 hours of life, whereby macromolecules such as immunoglobulins in colostrum are absorbed by pinocytosis, may also present a more permissive barrier to the uptake of MAP. The presence of anti-MAP antibodies in colostrum is not protective, and in fact, in 1 study, intestinal

The author has nothing to disclose.

Section of Large Animal Internal Medicine, Department of Clinical Studies–New Bolton Center, 382 West Street Road, Kennett Square, PA 19348, USA

E-mail address: rsweeney@vet.upenn.edu

doi:10.1016/j.cvfa.2011.07.001
0749-0720/11/$ – see front matter © 2011 Elsevier Inc. All rights reserved.
vetfood.theclinics.com

uptake of MAP was enhanced by opsonization with serum-derived antibodies against MAP.[10] Other hypotheses to explain the increased susceptibility of young calves relative to adults include possible immaturity of the innate or adaptive immune responses in young calves or the development of acquired immunity by adults as a result of exposure events that did not result in infection. Resistance of adult cattle to infection is most likely not due to a failure of MAP organisms to enter the tissues but rather to containment or elimination of MAP organisms once they penetrate the intestinal mucosa.[7–9]

In addition to the animal's age at exposure, the magnitude of the MAP dose ingested will also affect the course of the infection. In general, animals that ingest a higher dose of MAP will be more likely to become infected, and expected to progress to the clinical stage more rapidly, than those ingesting a lower dose. Age-related resistance to MAP may be overwhelmed if adult cattle are exposed to extremely contaminated environments. However, age-related resistance aside, cattle that ingest an infectious dose at an older age may be more likely to leave the herd because of culling due to other diseases or production-related culling before the long MAP incubation period is complete and Johne's disease is recognized.

In addition to the observation that resistance to infection with MAP increases with age, there has long been speculation that susceptibility to MAP may be genetically influenced. Evidence of genetic predisposition or resistance to MAP infection could include breed differences in susceptibility, association of MAP infection with certain family lines of cattle as determined by pedigree analysis or analysis of dam-daughter pairs, and, most recently, association of MAP infection with certain genotypes as determined by DNA analysis in infected versus uninfected cattle. Dating back to the earliest descriptions of Johne's disease in cattle, it has been speculated that the Channel Island breeds of cattle (Guernsey, Jersey) had a higher prevalence of Johne's disease and thus were more susceptible to MAP infection. However, it is not possible to determine whether these anecdotal observations represent a true genetic effect on susceptibility and to what extent management, geography, and other influences confound the observation.[11] Studies in beef cattle have suggested a higher prevalence of enzyme-linked immunosorbent assay (ELISA)–positive status among *Bos indicus* breeds compared with *Bos taurus* breeds[12] and that familial aggregates of ELISA-positive animals exist in Texas Longhorn cattle.[13] However, in those studies, infection with MAP was not confirmed by organism detection tests, and the effect of exposure to environmental mycobacteria on antibody status may have confounded the results. Analysis of familial associations based on dam-daughter pair observations may be confounded by increased opportunity for exposure in offspring of infected dams, either in utero, by colostrum, or direct contact. Studies that evaluate the influence of sire would not be confounded by these factors. These limitations aside, based on numerous published studies, the heritability of paratuberculosis in dairy cattle is estimated to be approximately 9% to 12%.[14] Heritability of MAP infection in Merino sheep was 18% in 1 study, compared with 7% in Romney sheep.[15] Specific genetic DNA markers associated with resistance have been studied with variable results, with most candidate genes studied to date not showing a significant association with MAP infection status. However, a recent study showed an association between MAP infection status and the *CARD15* (NOD2) gene, which was strongest in Brahman × Angus crossbred animals.[16] Similar results were not obtained when a population of Holstein cattle were studied.[14] Undoubtedly, additional studies of other candidate genes will shed further light on the specific mechanisms for inheritance of resistance to infection.

In summary, there is convincing evidence that genetic susceptibility may influence outcome of MAP exposure in cattle and sheep. However, at this time management and environmental factors are likely to outweigh genetic influences, but at some point genetic selection for increased resistance to infection may become a reality.

THE ORGANISM ENTERS

Once the animal is exposed orally to MAP, the organisms may invade via 2 separate portals of entry. Some early studies using experimental infections with large doses of MAP in calves showed that MAP likely invaded through the tonsils, with MAP organisms found in retropharyngeal lymphoid tissue shortly after exposure.[17] Direct inoculation of MAP into tonsillar crypts will also result in infection.[18] From there, the MAP organisms may spread either hematogenously or via lymph to mesenteric lymph nodes and ileum. However, most evidence, from experimental studies using less exaggerated doses of MAP, or homogenates of tissues from naturally infected cows, points to the ileum as the main portal of entry.[19–21] Specialized nonvillous epithelial cells located in the Peyer's patches of the small intestine, known as M cells, facilitate translocation of MAP across the intestinal epithelium. The MAP organisms are taken up by M cells and released on the submucosal side of the intestinal epithelium unchanged. Here the MAP organisms are scavenged by macrophages, which they enter via phagocytosis. Experimentally, MAP organisms were found within submucosal macrophages by 5 hours after direct inoculation into ileum of calves.[10]

At this point, the fate of the animal with respect to MAP infection is not yet sealed. If the macrophages are successful in killing the phagocytosed MAP organisms, then the infection might be thwarted. However, MAP organisms have a unique ability to survive within macrophages, and it is this characteristic that lies at the heart of the chronic progressive nature of paratuberculosis. Thus begins the protracted dance between host defenses and pathogen proliferation.

INFECTION BEGINS

As with most intracellular pathogens, macrophage killing of ingested MAP organisms is critical for the initial stage of host defense against establishment of a MAP infection. Macrophage activation by cytokines such as interferon-gamma, produced by Th1-type T-helper lymphocytes, enhances the killing of intracellular MAP organisms.[22] It is likely that some exposed cattle are successful in eliminating the MAP infection via this mechanism and thus do not progress to clinical Johne's disease. However, many exposed animals are unsuccessful at eliminating MAP, and the organism persists within macrophages in these animals. Although the mechanism for intracellular survival is not completely understood, MAP appears to prevent maturation and acidification of the phagocytic vacuole within the macrophage, thus preventing exposure of the MAP organisms to the bacteriocidal effects of lysozomal enzymes and oxygen-derived radicals.[23] Generally, early in infection, even in susceptible animals that will eventually succumb, the host defenses are able to contain the infection, allowing only slow proliferation and spread of MAP within the gut and gut-associated lymphoid tissue. This early, "controlled" infection results in an extended "eclipse phase" that may last for 2 or more years. During this time, the animal shows no outward clinical signs of infection, there is no appreciable effect on production or weight gain, and fecal shedding of MAP and serum antibodies are usually not detectable. Measures of specific cell-mediated immunity, such as in vitro assays that measure lymphocyte proliferation or production of interferon-gamma may yield positive results, but these tests are rarely practical in a clinical setting. The only reliable method to identify animals in this stage of infection is by sampling of ileum or mesenteric lymph node for MAP detection by culture or polymerase chain reaction.

Although the infection may be controlled in the early stages of infection, this occurs at some expense to the host. The presence of MAP antigens within intestinal submucosa and mesenteric lymph nodes incites an inflammatory response—the host's effort to contain the infection. Additional macrophages and lymphocytes are attracted to the area, and granuloma formation with multinucleated giant cells, epithelioid cells, lymphocytes, and macrophages ensues. In the early phase of infection, these lesions are limited in severity and localized, and in fact this response aids in the containment of MAP to the initial sites of infection.[24] Macrophages containing acid-fast organisms are sparse in these early, focal lesions. However, as the infection slowly progresses, the organism disseminates and the lesions become more severe, eventually manifesting as clinical disease. Thus, the granulomatous response initially contains the MAP infection, but the "collateral damage" caused by the granulomatous inflammation eventually leads to the clinical signs of Johne's disease.

INFECTION PROGRESSES

The granulomatous inflammatory response, while disrupting the mucosal structure and function particularly in the small intestine and associated lymph nodes, serves to confine MAP-laden macrophages to the gut and gut-associated lymphoid tissue. By this process, MAP and its host may coexist for many years, with no outward signs of disease in the host, yet all the while, MAP, despite being contained, is not killed. With time, and for reasons that are poorly understood, the infection begins to gain the upper hand. The cell-mediated immunity responsible for containing the infection begins to wane, and the infection begins to progress more rapidly. This loss of "control" of the infection is often associated with a transition from a Th1-type immune response where cytokines associated with macrophage activation (interferon-gamma) predominate, to a Th2-type immune response characterized by a predominance of cytokines such as IL-4 and IL-10, which are associated with onset of antibody production accompanied by waning of specific cell-mediated immunity.[25-27] The cause or trigger for the switch in the immune response is unknown, but as it occurs, infection progresses more rapidly,

With this loss of immune "control" of the infection, the infected animal begins to shed MAP in steadily increasing quantities in the feces, and MAP organisms spread to other tissues such as the uterus (causing in utero transmission), the mammary gland, and other internal organs and muscle tissue.[1-4] At this stage, the animal may still not be showing any outward clinical signs of disease, and in most cases, development of antibodies detectable by ELISA will not occur until after fecal shedding has begun.[28]

Although these animals do not show outward clinical signs of Johne's disease, studies have shown a reduction in milk production may occur up to 300 days before the animal produces antibodies to MAP detectable by ELISA.[29] Reduction in milk production up to 16% compared to uninfected animals is seen in the final lactation before culling, and in 1 study, a 4% reduction in the penultimate lactation was found, an effect that was not observed in all studies.[30-32] Similarly, cows that are in this subclinical stage of the infection may have reduced reproductive efficiency. In a recent study, days open was increased by 28 days for ELISA-positive cows compared with ELISA-negative cows in the same herds. However, when cows' infection status was classified by fecal culture results, there was no difference on days open associated with MAP infection.[33] Other studies have reported no significant effect on reproductive efficiency.[32] Using milk somatic cell count or linear score as a measure of udder health, reports have been mixed, with some showing a negative effect, some no effect, and some even a positive effect on udder health.[32]

Clearly, in the subclinical stage of MAP infection where fecal shedding and antibody production have begun, there may be an effect on production efficiency but it may not be easily identified by the producer.

CLINICAL DISEASE BEGINS

Eventually, after fecal shedding of MAP and serum antibodies are detectable, overt clinical signs of Johne's disease become apparent. Just as the time from onset of infection to first detectable fecal shedding of MAP is quite variable (but usually > 2 years), the duration of the asymptomatic fecal shedder stage is quite variable. Some cattle progress rapidly to the clinical stage, in some cases within 6 months of first fecal shedding, and in some cases asymptomatic fecal shedding continues for several years without cattle progressing to clinical disease.

As the MAP infection progresses, the lesions in the intestines and mesenteric lymph nodes become more severe. Rather than focal or multifocal lesions, the granulomatous infiltrate becomes diffuse, affecting jejunum, ileum, cecum, and, to a lesser extent, colon. The lining of the small intestine, particularly the ileum, becomes thickened due to the massive cellular infiltration (**Fig. 1**), and the intestinal villi become "clubbed" or shortened and thickened, reducing their absorptive effectiveness (**Fig. 2**). Granulomatous lymphadenitis leads to lymphangectasia, and rupture of lacteals with fistulation into the bowel lumen. In cattle, macrophages laden with MAP organisms generally are abundant within the lesions.[21,24]

The granulomatous inflammation centered on the ileum but also involving other segments of small and large intestine, causes malabsorption, diarrhea, and protein losing enteropathy with hypoproteinemia. The hallmark clinical sign in cattle is watery ("pipe-stream") diarrhea. The feces do not have grossly visible blood or mucus, and the cows do not exhibit tenesmus. Despite the watery feces, cows do not become dehydrated, although increased water consumption may occur to compensate for the excessive fecal water lost. Vital signs are normal, and the cow's appetite remains good until the terminal stages of the disease. In some instances, in the early clinical

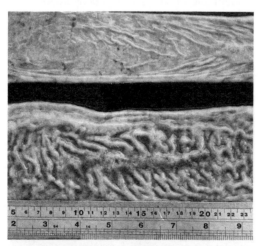

Fig. 1. Ileum from a cow with clinical Johne's disease (*bottom*), demonstrating thickening of the mucosa and prominent Peyer's patches, compared with ileum from a normal cow (*top*). (*Courtesy of* Michael T. Collins, DVM, PhD, Madison, WI.)

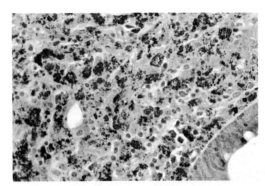

Fig. 2. Histopathologic section of ileum (acid-fast stain) from a cow with paratuberculosis demonstrating intracellular acid-fast organisms. (*Courtesy of* Michael T. Collins, DVM, PhD, Madison, WI.)

stages of the disease, the feces may return to normal consistency for several weeks or months, and then diarrhea may again resume. Anecdotally, clinical signs of Johne's disease may be exacerbated following the stress of parturition and early lactation, but attempts to precipitate clinical signs with corticosteroid administration have generally not been successful. Weight loss usually accompanies the diarrhea (**Fig. 3**), and as the plasma protein concentration falls, subcutaneous edema may develop, especially in dependent areas such as the brisket or submandibular area ("bottle jaw") (**Fig. 4**). Milk production is reduced by 20% or more, and in terminal stages may be nearly zero. In this advanced stage of disease, metastasis of MAP organisms to extraintestinal sites occurs frequently, and fetal infection in utero occurs in 40% or more of these cases.[1] Massive fecal shedding of MAP by clinically affected animals results in significant environmental contamination. Most animals are culled once the typical clinical signs are recognized but, if allowed to remain in the herd, will progress to a moribund state with death due to cachexia and dehydration.

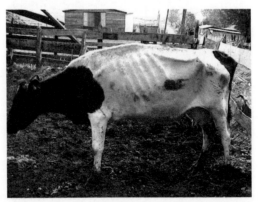

Fig. 3. A Holstein cow with clinical paratuberculosis exhibiting marked weight loss. (*Courtesy of* Michael T. Collins, DVM, PhD, Madison, WI.)

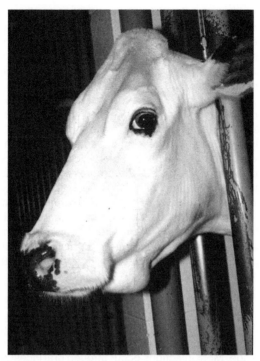

Fig. 4. Submandibular edema ("bottle jaw") in a cow with clinical paratuberculosis and hypoproteinemia. (*Courtesy of* Michael T. Collins, DVM, PhD, Madison, WI.)

PARATUBERCULOSIS IN NONBOVIDS

A wide range of host species beyond cattle, including sheep, goats, camelids, and deer, among others are susceptible to MAP infection. In general, the pathogenesis of infection in these species is similar to that in cattle, with early occult infection eventually progressing to loss of immune control, with increasing bacterial burden and eventual clinical signs. However, there are some notable differences in the susceptibility, progression, characteristic pathologic lesions, and clinical signs among the various hosts.

The pathogenesis and progression of MAP infection in sheep have been particularly well studied. As with cattle, infection was thought to occur early in life, with lambs being most susceptible. However, as with cattle, it appears that age-related resistance can be overcome if MAP exposure is heavy. A recent longitudinal study that involved sequential intestinal and mesenteric lymph node biopsies in naturally exposed sheep raised under routine production conditions revealed that new infections occurred at a steady rate between the ages of 9 months and 36 months under conditions of continuous or repeated exposure.[34] In sheep, a paucibacillary form of infection, characterized by lymphocytic infiltration and few acid-fast bacteria, is described, often compared with the tuberculoid form of leprosy. This form of infection has been associated with a Th1-type immune response, which favors cell-mediated immune control of the MAP infection.[35] Sheep with paucibacillary enteritis may progress to multibacillary enteritis (characterized by numerous acid-fast organisms, macrophages, and granulomatous reaction, or lepromatous form) or, in some instances, may recover.[34]

Clinical signs in small ruminants and alpacas, which normally have pelleted feces, may be less apparent because diarrhea, although possible, is less commonly seen compared with cattle. Feces may lose their normal pelleted conformation, assuming a consistency more similar to dog feces, or the feces may remain normal. Thus, in many small ruminant cases, weight loss, hypoproteinemia, and edema are the most common clinical findings, and intestinal parasitism is often the initial suspected cause. Additionally, in the author's experience, goats with Johne's disease are often anemic, more severe than one might normally expect from anemia of chronic disease, although that is the suspected cause of anemia in those cases.

The pathogenesis and clinical progression of paratuberculosis in farmed deer also differ from those in cattle and small ruminants. As with cattle, young deer appear more susceptible than yearlings or adults, but the progression of disease appears much more rapid in young deer compared with cattle. Clinical signs may progress over a period of a few weeks and include loose feces and unthrifty condition.[36] Pathologic lesions also differ from cattle, in that caseation or calcification of enlarged mesenteric lymph nodes may be seen resulting in lesions indistinguishable from tuberculosis. As with sheep, both paucibacillary and multibacillary forms of infection are seen.[36] The frequency of transplacental infection in deer, which approaches 90%, is also higher than that reported for cattle or sheep.[37]

SUMMARY

MAP is a hearty intracellular pathogen that can persist in the environment for long periods of time. Animals are generally most susceptible in the neonatal period and gain resistance with age. Most infections occur through oral ingestion of MAP shed in the feces of adult animals, but in utero transmission can also occur. Ingested MAP organisms are able to survive within host macrophages. Initially, host immune defenses are able to control proliferation of the organisms, resulting in a prolonged period of incubation during which there are no clinical signs. However, during this "eclipse" phase, a destructive granulomatous inflammatory response develops that eventually leads to intestinal malabsorption and protein losing enteropathy. In the final stages of the infection, decreased production, weight loss, diarrhea, and hypoproteinemia are present, despite a good appetite. Fecal shedding occurs before other clinical signs, so that asymptomatic carrier animals may contaminate premises and infect susceptible animals before it is known that they are infectious.

REFERENCES

1. Streeter RN, Hoffsis GF, Bech-Nielsen S, et al. Isolation of Mycobacterium paratuberculosis from colostrum and milk of subclinically infected cows. Am J Vet Res 1995; 56:1322–4.
2. Sweeney RW, Whitlock RH, Rosenberger AE. Mycobacterium paratuberculosis cultured from milk and supramammary lymph nodes of infected asymptomatic cows. J Clin Microbiol 1992;30:166–71.
3. Seitz SE, Heider LE, Hueston WD, et al. Bovine fetal infection with Mycobacterium paratuberculosis. J Am Vet Med Assoc 1989;194:1423–6.
4. Sweeney RW, Whitlock RH, Rosenberger AE. Mycobacterium paratuberculosis isolated from fetuses of infected cows not manifesting signs of the disease. Am J Vet Res 1992;53:477–80.
5. Hagan WA. Age as a factor in susceptibility to Johne's disease. Cornell Vet 1938;28: 34–40.
6. Rankin JD. Experimental infection. Vet Rec 1959;71:1157–67.

7. Payne JM, Rankin JD. A comparison of the pathogenesis of experimental Johne's disease in calves and cows. Res Vet Sci 1961;2:175–9.

8. Rankin JD. The experimental infection of cattle with *Mycobacterium johnei*. J Comp Pathol 1961;71:6–9.

9. Larsen AB, Merkal RS, Cutlip RC. Age of cattle related to resistance to infection with *Mycobacterium paratuberculosis*. Am J Vet Res 1975;36:255–7.

10. Momotani E, Whipple DL, Thiermann AB, et al. Role of M cells in the entrance of *Mycobacterium paratuberculosis* into domes of ileal Peyers patches in calves. Vet Pathol 1988;25:131–7.

11. Chiodini RJ, van Kruiningen HJ, Merkal RS. Ruminant paratuberculosis (Johne's disease): the current status and future prospects. Cornell Vet 1984;74:218–62.

12. Roussel AJ, Libal MC, Whitlock RH, et al. Prevalence of and risk factors for paratuberculosis in purebred beef cattle. J Am Vet Med Assoc 2005;226:773–6.

13. Ostertock JB, Fosgate GT, Derr JN, et al. Assessing familial aggregation of paratuberculosis in beef cattle of unknown pedigree. Prev Vet Med 2008;84:121–34.

14. Kirkpatrick BW. Genetics of host susceptibility to paratuberculosis. In: Behr MA, Collins DM, editors. Pararuberculosis: organism, disease, control. Oxfordshire, UK: CABI International; 2010. p. 50–9.

15. Hickey SM, Morris CA, Dobbie JL, et al. Heritability of Johne's disease and survival data from Romney and Merino sheep. Proc N Z Soc Anim Prod 2003;63:179–82.

16. Pinedo PJ, Buergelt CD, Donovan GA, et al. Association between CARD15/NOD2 gene polymorphisms and paratuberculosis infection in cattle. Vet Microbiol 2009;134: 346–52.

17. Payne JM, Rankin JD. The pathogenesis of experimental Johne's disease in calves. Res Vet Sci 1961;2:167–74.

18. Waters WR, Miller JM, Palmer MC, et al. Early induction of humoral and cellular immune responses during experimental *Mycobacterium avium* subsp. *paratuberculosis* infection of calves. Infect Immun 2003;71:5130–8.

19. Gilmour NJL, Nisbet DI, Brotherston JG. Experimental oral infection of calves with *Mycobacterium johnei*. J Comp Pathol 1965;75:281–6.

20. Sweeney RW, Uzonna J, Whitlock RH, et al. Tissue predilection sites and effect of dose on *Mycobacterium avium* subsp. *paratuberculosis* organism recovery in a short-term bovine experimental oral infection model. Res Vet Sci 2006;80:253–9.

21. Buergelt CD, Hall C, McEntee K, et al. Pathologic evaluation of paratuberculosis in naturally infected cattle. Vet Pathol 1978;15:196–207.

22. Zurbrick BG, Follett DM, Czuprynski CJ. Cytokine regulation of the intracellular growth of *Mycobacterium paratuberculosis* in bovine monocytes. Infect Immun 1988;56: 1692–7.

23. Hostetter J, Steadham E, Haynes J, et al. Phagosomal maturation and intracellular survival of *Mycobacterium avium* subspecies *paratuberculosis* in J774 cells. Comp Immunology Microbiol Infect Dis 2003;26:269–83.

24. Gonzalez J, Geijo MV, Garcia-Pariente C. Histopathologic classification of lesions associated with natural paratuberculosis infection in cattle. J Comp Pathol 2005;133: 184–96.

25. Stabel JR. Cytokine secretion by peripheral blood mononuclear cells from cows infected with *Mycobacterium paratuberculosis*. Am J Vet Res 2000;61:754–60.

26. Sweeney RW, Jones DE, Habecker P, et al. Interferon-gamma and interleukin-4 gene expression in cows infected with *Mycobacterium paratuberculosis*. Am J Vet Res 1998;59:842–7.

27. Stabel JR. Transitions in immune responses to *Mycobacterium paratuberculosis*. Vet Microbiol 2000;77:465–73.

28. Sweeney RW, Whitlock RH, McAdams S, et al. Longitudinal study of ELISA reactivity to *Mycobacterium avium* subsp. *paratuberculosis* in infected cattle and culture negative herd mates. J Vet Diagn Invest 2006;18:2–6.

29. Nielsen SS, Krogh MA, Enevoldsen C. Time to the occurrence of a decline in milk production in cows with various paratuberculosis antibody profiles. J Dairy Sci 2009;92:149–55.

30. Benedictus G, Dijkhuizen AA, Stelwagen J. Economic losses due to paratuberculosis in dairy cattle. Vet Rec 1987;121:142–6.

31. Lombard JE, Garry FB, McCluskey BJ, et al. Risk of removal and effects on milk production associated with paratuberculosis status in dairy herds. J Am Vet Med Assoc 2005;227:1975–81.

32. Gonda MG, Chang YM, Shook GE, et al. Effect of *Mycobacterium paratuberculosis* infection on production, reproduction, and health traits in US cattle. Prev Vet Med 2007;80:103–19.

33. Johnson-Ifearulundu YJ, Kaneene JB, Sprecher DJ, et al. The effect of subclinical *Mycobacterium paratuberculosis* infection on days open in Michigan, USA dalry cow. Prev Vet Med 2000;46:171–81.

34. Dennis MM, Reddacliff LA, Whittington RJ. Longitudinal study of clinicopathological features of Johne's disease in sheep naturally exposed to *Mycobacterium avium* subspecies *paratuberculosis*. Vet Pathol 2011;48:565–75.

35. Perez V, Tellechea J, Corpra JM, et al. Relation between pathologic findings and cellular immune responses in sheep with naturally acquired paratuberculosis. Am J Vet Res 1999;60:123–7.

36. Mackintosh CG, Griffin JF. Pararuberculosis in deer, camelids, and other ruminants. In: Behr MA, Collins DM, editors. Pararuberculosis: organism, disease, control. Oxfordshire, UK: CABI International; 2010. p. 180–7.

37. van Kooten HCJ, Mackintonsh CG, Koets AP. Intra-uterine transmission of paratuberculosis (Johne's disease) in farmed deer. N Z Vet J 2006;54:16–20.

Treatment and Chemoprophylaxis for Paratuberculosis

Marie-Eve Fecteau, DVM*, Robert H. Whitlock, DVM, PhD

KEYWORDS

- Johne's disease • Paratuberculosis • Treatment
- Chemoprophylaxis • Cattle • Ruminants

There are no definitive cures for *Mycobacterium avium* subsp. *paratuberculosis* (MAP) infections, but several therapeutic agents may be employed to reduce or alleviate the clinical signs (mainly weight loss and diarrhea) associated with MAP infections and help prolong the life of the animal. Treatment typically must be maintained for the life of the animal and treated animals usually continue to shed MAP organisms, but often in reduced numbers. In addition, there are currently no drugs approved for paratuberculosis treatment in food producing animals in the United States. However, therapeutic options do exist for cattle and other ruminants that are of significant economic, genetic or sentimental value. Occasionally, veterinarians will be asked to treat animals with Johne's disease (JD) that are pets or used for sport, such as bulls in rodeo events. Owners who are financially able to house and maintain MAP-infected cattle or other ruminants without being able to sell the meat or milk for human consumption may consider treatment of their animals.

Published reports on the treatment of cattle with JD have focused on the preservation of genetic material (embryos and semen), not on the salvage of the carcass for meat or milk production.[1–3] In all situations, drugs used in the treatment of JD would be used in an "extra-label" manner with the veterinarian responsible for providing guidelines to the owner about milk and meat withdrawal times. The authors strongly advise that owners of animals being treated for JD sign a statement that the milk and meat from the animal will *never* be used for human consumption. This statement will at least demonstrate that the owner was informed about the animal's use for food production.

The authors have nothing to disclose.
Department of Clinical Studies–New Bolton Center, School of Veterinary Medicine, University of Pennsylvania, 382 West Street Road, Kennett Square, PA 19348, USA
* Corresponding author.
E-mail address: mfecteau@vet.upenn.edu

Vet Clin Food Anim 27 (2011) 547–557
doi:10.1016/j.cvfa.2011.07.002
0749-0720/11/$ – see front matter © 2011 Elsevier Inc. All rights reserved.

DEFINITIVE DIAGNOSIS

Other diseases of cattle, such as renal amyloidosis, severe parasitism, intestinal neoplasia, and post caval thrombosis, may result in weight loss and chronic diarrhea that mimic clinical signs of JD.[4] Therefore, prior to treatment of a JD-suspect animal, the veterinarian is obligated to establish a definitive diagnosis of MAP infection using reliable diagnostic procedures such as culture, reverse transcription–polymerase chain reaction, or histology of the ileum and/or ileocecal lymph node.

EDUCATION OF THE OWNER

Once a definitive diagnosis has been established, the owner needs to be fully informed about the implications of keeping an animal with clinical JD on the premises. These animals are in the advanced stage of the infection, shedding millions of MAP per day and making transmission to susceptible animals likely. Therefore, it is recommended that these animals be moved to a location well away from susceptible animals.

Reports of animals treated for JD indicate that they may clinically recover and regain body weight and normal fecal consistency, although there is limited evidence of a true bacteriologic cure of MAP infections in animals.[1–3,5–9] Treatment may substantially reduce MAP fecal shedding, sometimes leading to low-level shedding or even negative fecal cultures in some animals.[1] However, tissues from treated animals remain infected with viable MAP.[1,10]

In cases of disseminated MAP infections, nongastrointestinal tissues including reproductive organs such as the epididymis, testes and seminal vesicles in males, and uterine mucosa in cows may also be infected.[11–14] Most commercial artificial insemination centers require bulls to be test-negative for MAP, making treatment of valuable bulls kept for breeding rarely justified. The most recent literature estimated that 9% of fetuses born from subclinically infected dams and 39% of clinically affected dams were infected in utero with MAP.[15] Therefore, treated cows that become pregnant have a risk of in utero fetal infection and the authors advise against keeping offspring of clinically affected dams, even if treated, within the herd. Alternatives such as supra-ovulation, in vitro fertilization, and cloning are available today to help preserve the genetic potential of prized animals. While an embryo obtained from a cow with a disseminated MAP infection could result in an infected fetus, the risk is deemed very low.[15,16] This practice is also considered safe for the recipient cow.[17] If the decision is made to treat an animal with JD, treatment should be continued for several weeks before collecting embryos or semen to allow the animal to regain weight, and be in a positive energy and protein balance. In addition, little is known regarding the effects of drugs used for treatment of JD on semen and embryos. Isoniazid and clofazimine have been shown to have feticidal effect in laboratory animals and are not recommended for use during pregnancy in humans.[18] Possible side effects of each of the drugs are discussed in more detail later.

TREATMENT OPTIONS

Because MAP grows intracellularly, most drugs used for treatment of JD are able to penetrate mammalian cells and many of those drugs have been derived from therapies for tuberculosis in humans. Antimicrobials that have been used in experimental and natural cases of paratuberculosis in animals include isoniazid, rifampin, clofazimine, aminoglycosides, and dapsone.[1–3,6,9,19] Most reports concerning tuberculosis therapy in humans suggest drug combinations are superior to monotherapy.[20]

Combinations of antimicrobials have been used to treat cattle, goats, and laboratory animals.[3,9,19] There are insufficient data available with which to judge the frequency of drug resistance among strains of MAP, but resistance occurs to virtually all available drugs used to treat human tuberculosis.

Isoniazid

Isoniazid (isonicotinic acid), inhibits biosynthesis of mycolic acids, a major component of the mycobacterial cell wall.[21] It is bactericidal for the first 2 days of treatment when mycobacteria are rapidly growing and then bacteriostatic for the remainder of the therapy when the pathogen's replication rate has slowed.[21] Pharmacokinetic studies in ruminants indicate that it is well absorbed orally, diffuses well to body fluids, and penetrate cells easily.[22,23]

Isoniazid, one of the earliest drugs used to treat cattle with JD, has been used for several decades to treat human tuberculosis. Two of the earliest reports on isoniazid treatment of JD and prevention of MAP infections in experimentally challenged calves failed to provide evidence of efficacy.[5,24] Later, Baldwin reported the successful treatment of JD in a cow using 11 mg/kg.[25] In that report, the cow's appetite improved within 7 days of treatment initiation and weight gain began after 2 weeks.[25] Another report provides evidence of clinical efficacy in 2 isoniazid-treated cows (11 mg/kg) when used in combination with rifampin (22 mg/kg), gentamicin (2.2 mg/kg), and ampicillin (11 mg/kg).[3] The 2 cows described in that case report were maintained on isoniazid for nearly 2 years using a 3 weeks on/1 week off treatment protocol. One of the 2 cows remained in complete clinical remission while the other had intermittent periods of weight loss and diarrhea. These reports illustrate that treatment of clinical cases of JD with isoniazid alone or in combination with other antimicrobials may induce clinical remission but does not eliminate the MAP infection.

Plasma levels of 2 to 5 μg/mL are required to slow MAP growth.[24] The minimum recommended dose is 11 mg/kg while a higher dose of 25 mg/kg was well tolerated by cattle experimentally treated for a total of 11 weeks.[26] Isoniazid is metabolized by the liver and can cause hepatic damage characterized histopathologically by bridging and multilobular necrosis.[27] When administered to cattle at 30 mg/kg, toxicity signs include feed refusal, decreased milk production, and rear limb stiffness.[22,23] Severe ataxia may occur at 60 mg/kg and death at 100 mg/kg.[23] Thus the recommended dose for treatment of animals with JD is 20 mg/kg orally once a day and periodic assessment of liver function is recommended. No congenital anomalies due to isoniazid have been reported in mice, rabbits, or rats at recommended doses.[25] However, practitioners should be aware of the possibility of the drug inducing abortion in cattle.[28,29]

Rifampin

Rifampin, a semisynthetic antibiotic derived from rifamycin B, has a broad antimicrobial spectrum of action and is either bactericidal or bacteriostatic depending on the test organism and concentration of the drug. Rifampin enters leukocytes and is therefore particularly efficacious against intracellular microorganisms, being routinely used for the treatment of human tuberculosis, equine *Rhodococcus equi* infections, and internal abscesses in animals.[30,31]

Growth of *M. tuberculosis* in vitro was inhibited by rifampin at concentrations of 0.005 μg/mL to 0.2 μg/mL.[30] The MIC of rifampin for 12 MAP strains (7 human-origin and 5 animal-origin) was between 0.5 μg/mL and greater than 2 μg/mL.[32] In vitro, combinations of 6-mercaptopurine-rifampicin and arithromycin-rifampicin were synergistic when tested against 4 of 9 tested MAP isolates.[33]

It is recommended that rifampin always be administered concurrently with another antimicrobial agent because of drug synergy and to decrease the potential for drug resistance development. Following experimental infection with MAP, rabbits treated with a combination of streptomycin (10 mg/kg twice daily) and rifampin (10 mg/kg once daily), in combination with levamisole, not only regained body weight and normal fecal consistency, but their intestinal tissues were culture-negative for MAP at postmortem examination.[34] The same researchers also found that treatment with a rifampin-levamisole combination was superior to a streptomycin-levamisole combination.[34] In another report of naturally occurring JD in a goat, treatment with streptomycin-isoniazid-rifampin successfully alleviated the clinical signs of diarrhea and weight loss, and culture of tissues obtained at necropsy (85 days into treatment) were negative for MAP growth.[9]

Rifampin is absorbed orally in ruminants,[35,36] and pharmacokinetic data indicate a dosage of 20 mg/kg orally every 24 hours should provide adequate serum concentrations for treatment of rifampin-sensitive bacterial infections.[35,36] The most frequent side effects in humans relate to renal failure and have been associated with the administration of large doses of the drug. Adverse side effects have not been reported with its use in foals, adult horses, sheep, or cattle.[35,36] A major obstacle to the use of rifampin in cattle remains its cost.

Clofazimine

Clofazimine, a phenazine iminoquinone derivative, was first used in the treatment of sulfone resistant leprosy.[37] Its mode of action is to bind to and inhibit the template function of bacterial DNA.[38] Clofazimine accumulates in fat tissue and in the macrophages of the reticuloendothelial system and thus has good efficacy against intracellular pathogens such as MAP.[6]

Three early reports on clofazimine indicated significant beneficial effects on experimental MAP infections in young lambs.[6–8] Lambs treated with 15 mg/kg of clofazimine and challenged weekly for 10 weeks with 10^8 MAP organisms[6] had reduced infection rates of mesenteric lymph nodes but not intestinal mucosa.[6] The administration of clofazimine at the same dose to lambs with established MAP infections resulted in a reduced number of organisms in the intestinal tract and mesenteric lymph nodes but did not completely eliminate the infection.[6] Treated sheep had orange pigmentation of fat but no other signs of toxicity.[6] One report described a favorable clinical response in 2 naturally MAP-infected cows treated with 2 mg/kg of clofazimine for 200 days and 330 days, respectively.[1] In both cows, MAP fecal shedding levels decreased greatly and the animals returned to normal health.[1] The cow treated for 200 days relapsed after discontinuation of treatment. Both cows had MAP culture-positive tissues at necropsy.[1] In another report on the clofazimine treatment of naturally MAP-infected cows, a clinical response was seen (weight gain, increase in plasma protein concentration, and improved manure consistency) in cows receiving 600 mg/day of clofazimine.[2] Fecal cultures, however, remained positive for MAP. The authors' conclusion was that clofazimine does not completely eliminate the infection but can alleviate clinical signs of JD when the cows are kept on the drug for the reminder of the lives.[2] No signs of toxicity were seen in the studies reported here.[1,2]

The authors recommend 600 to 1000 mg of clofazimine orally daily for the reminder of the cow's life. Clinical response, with reduction in severity of diarrhea and resolution of submandibular edema, is often apparent within a few days of starting treatment. Total plasma protein concentration typically begins to increase within 1 to 2 weeks, and weight gain is obvious within a month. Cessation of treatment typically results in relapse within 7 to 14 days. A major problem with clofazimine use is its lack of availability in the United States. However, the drug may be imported from other countries such as Canada.

Other Treatment Options

A number of aminoglycosides (streptomycin, kanamycin, gentamicin, and amikacin) are active against several species of mycobacteria, including MAP.[30,39–41] More recently, newer drugs including cyclosporine A, rapamycin, tacrolimus, 5-aminosalicyclic acid, methotrexate, azathioprine, and its metabolite 6-mercaptopurine have been evaluated in vitro against several strains of MAP.[32,33,42–45] Interest in the efficacy of these drugs against MAP stems from the possible link between MAP and Crohn's disease.[46] To avoid use of human drugs in animals and for economic reasons, use of these drugs in food producing animals may not be appropriate.

In one case report, levamisole was administered intramuscularly to 19 MAP ELISA-positive cows at a dose of 2.5 mg/kg once daily for 3 days then once weekly for 8 weeks.[47] Treatment resulted in fewer acid-fast bacilli in fecal samples of the levamisole-treated cows compared to placebo controls.[47] Levamisole is thought to act as an immunomodulator boosting cell-mediated immunity via the induction of type 1 cytokines.[48,49]

The antimicrobial activity of certain naturally occurring compounds has long been demonstrated.[50] A recent publication explored the in vitro antibacterial activity of 18 naturally occurring compounds against MAP find that 6 of 18 compounds tested, including trans-cinnamaldehyde, cinnamon oil, oregano oil, and carvacrol, inhibited MAP growth.[51] As research about natural products progresses, findings applicable to the veterinary field may become available.

Recently, probiotics have been used in both human and veterinary medicine as potential therapeutic agents for a variety of diseases. One agent, Dietzia subsp C79793-74, was reported to inhibit MAP growth under specific in vitro conditions and has been evaluated in the treatment of paratuberculosis in cattle.[52–54] MAP test-positive cows given daily doses of Dietzia subsp, typically top-dressed on the feed, had statistically significant longer survival times compared to MAP test-positive control cows.[53] Of the Dietzia-treated MAP test-positive cows, 6 of 16 showed declining ELISA test scores overtime and became ELISA negative by the end of the study period, although this was not significantly different from controls.[53] In a larger follow-up study, the researchers found similar results and concluded that (1) Dietzia treatment resulted in a longitudinal decline in ELISA values; (2) Dietzia treatment was associated with a prolonged survival time; and (3) Dietzia-treated animals were the only ones to "cure" the disease.[54] More and independent research is needed substantiate the efficacy of Dietzia for treatment or control of paratuberculosis.

CHEMOPROPHYLAXIS

It is generally accepted that most calves become infected with MAP very early in life.[17] For this reason, control programs are primarily based on preventing direct or indirect MAP transmission from adult cattle to young replacement stock raised on the farm. Vaccination, available on a limited basis in the United States, may reduce the incidence of clinical disease and was associated with reduced colonization of intestinal tissues in experimental studies, but vaccinates are not fully protected from infection and can still shed MAP in their feces.[55–57] Prophylactic administration of an antimicrobial agent to neonatal calves during the period of high susceptibility and high exposure risk may represent an additional approach to MAP infection prevention.

Monensin

Monensin (Rumensin), an ionophore, has been widely used in the beef industry for years to enhance feed efficiency and to control coccidiosis.[58,59] More recently, monensin has been used in dairy cattle to improve energy metabolism and milk production and to alter milk components.[60] Monensin is a carboxylic polyether ionophore produced by Streptomyces cinnamonensis and is fed to cattle as a sodium salt.[61] It binds to bacterial cell membranes, especially those of gram-positive bacteria including Mycobacteria, causing an efflux of potassium and an influx of hydrogen ions into the cell.[62] The cell expends energy to maintain the electrochemical gradient resulting in death or reduced growth of the affected bacteria.

Brumbaugh and collaborators first demonstrated a reduction in the number of colony-forming units of MAP from the livers of experimentally infected mice treated with 15 and 30 mg/kg of monensin compared to nontreated controls.[63] The MIC of monensin for 1 field isolate of MAP was found to be 0.39 μg/mL.[64] A subsequent in vitro study showed dose-dependent growth inhibition for 5 MAP strains.[65] A field trial on cattle naturally MAP-infected and fed monensin (450 mg daily) for 120 days demonstrated reduced severity of MAP-related histological lesions in the liver, ileum, and rectal mucosa (but not mesenteric lymph nodes) compared to controls.[66]

In a study of nearly 5000 Canadian dairy cows in 94 herds, monensin usage was associated with reduced occurrence of MAP milk-ELISA positivity.[67] In 48 herds where JD had not been detected previously and in another group of 46 herds where paratuberculosis had been detected previously, monensin use was associated with a reduced odds ratio of a cow testing positive for MAP infection by the milk-ELISA.[67] Monensin usage included both monensin premix and controlled release capsules (CRCs).[67] In another study that used CRC boluses designed to release 335 mg monensin per day in MAP fecal culture-positive dairy cows, treated cows had a moderate decrease in MAP fecal colony counts during the 98-day study period.[68]

Monensin was evaluated for MAP infection prevention on 12 neonatal Holstein calves. Six calves received 35 mg of monensin added to the milk replacer at each twice-a-day feeding for a total of 70 mg of monensin/treated calf/day.[69] The other 6 calves served as placebo controls. Both groups were challenged with 2 oral doses of cultured MAP cells on 2 consecutive days between days 7 and 9 of the trial. At the time of challenge, the calves were between 8 and 11 days of age. Calves were euthanized between days 65 and 67 days after starting the trial. Feces and 50 individual tissues, including multiple sections of intestine, abdominal organs, and mesenteric and peripheral lymph nodes, were harvested from each calf and processed for MAP isolation by culture on solid medium (HEYM). Calves fed monensin had fewer culture-positive fecal samples and fewer MAP colony-forming units detected in their manure compared to controls. Furthermore, monensin-fed calves had fewer culture-positive tissues and lower numbers of MAP in their tissues compared to controls. Results of this study suggested that monensin effectively reduced tissue colonization with MAP following oral challenge and reduced MAP fecal shedding.[69–70] Presumably, reduced tissue colonization in this short-term model translates to a lower likelihood of MAP shedding in manure and clinical disease in adulthood.[69] It should be noted that monensin was found to be relatively insoluble in milk. Therefore, the authors recommend thorough and constant mixing if monensin is added to milk fed to calves.

Monensin is safe when used in target species and at the recommended dosages.[71] Intoxication may come after mixing errors that result in its inclusion in the diets of nontarget species or in excessive concentrations in the diets of target species.[72] The toxicity of monensin in cattle and other species is known to be dose dependent.[73] In cattle, the clinical signs of acute monensin toxicity are anorexia (24 to 36 hours post ingestion), diarrhea, dullness, weakness, ataxia, dyspnea, prostration, and death within 3 to 14 days post ingestion of the incriminated feed.[74] Typical pathological findings in cattle suffering from monensin toxicity are cardiac and skeletal muscle degeneration and necrosis, with secondary lesions resulting from acute cardiac failure or chronic cardiovascular insufficiency.[74]

In conclusion, monensin added to cattle rations at all phases of their life may supplement MAP control by management practices at the farm level through enhanced infection resistance of calves and diminished MAP shedding by adult cattle lowering the MAP bioburden on the farm.

Gallium

Gallium (Ga) is a trivalent semimetal that shares many similarities with ferric iron and functions as an iron mimic. Ga is preferentially taken up by phagocytes at sites of inflammation, and its biologic effect on susceptible microorganisms appears related to its ability to substitute for ferric iron in many cellular metabolic pathways and disrupt them.[75,76] The in vitro antimicrobial activity of Ga has been shown against various microorganisms, including *Rhodococcus equi*, *Pseudomonas aeruginosa*, *Mycobacterium tuberculosis*, and *Mycobacterium avium* complex.[76–78] More recently, the authors demonstrated the in vitro antimicrobial efficacy of Ga against 10 MAP isolates.[79] In a follow-up experiment using Ga in neonatal calves experimentally challenged with MAP, the authors found that (1) Ga treatment was associated with a significant reduction in MAP tissue burden compared to controls and (2) no adverse effects related to Ga were seen in the treated calves.[80] Further studies are needed to determine the optimal chemoprophylactic dose of Ga for neonatal calves or therapeutic value for adult cattle. Additional concerns regarding use of Ga in cattle include drug residues, cost, and environmental impact.

SUMMARY

There is no definitive cure for infections with MAP, but a number of therapeutic agents may be employed to reduce or alleviate the clinical signs of JD and help prolong the life of cattle and other ruminants that are of significant economic, genetic, or sentimental value. Treatment typically must be maintained for the life of the animal and treated animals usually continue to shed MAP. In addition, there are currently no drugs approved for treatment of MAP infections in food producing animals in the United States; therefore, any drug use is done "extra-label." Drugs most commonly used for treatment of JD in ruminants include isoniazid, rifampin, and clofazimine.

JD control programs are primarily based on preventing direct or indirect transmission of MAP organisms from adult cattle to young replacement stock on the farm. Prophylactic administration of an antimicrobial agent to neonatal calves during the period of high susceptibility and high exposure risk may represent an additional approach to the prevention of MAP infections. Monensin, added to cattle rations at all phases of their life, may play a useful role both in the prevention of MAP infections in young cattle and to diminish fecal shedding by infected adults. Gallium as a chemoprophylactic agent against MAP in neonatal calves and has shown promising results.

REFERENCES

1. Merkal RS, Larsen AB. Clofazimine treatment of cows naturally infected with *Mycobacterium paratuberculosis*. Am J Vet Res 1973;34:27–8.

2. Whitlock RH, Divers T, Palmer J, et al. Johne's disease: A case study with clofazimine therapy in a dairy cow. In: Proceedings of the International Colloquium for Research on Paratuberculosis, 1983. p. 231–7.

3. Hoffsis GF, Streeter RN, Rings DM, et al. Therapy for Johne's disease. Bovine Pract 1990;25:55–8.

4. Roussel AJ, Whitlock RH. Chronic diarrhea in cattle: Differential diagnosis. In: Proceedings of the 14th World Congress on Diseases of Cattle. Dublin, 1986. p. 307–18.

5. Larsen AB, Vardamam TH. The effect of isonicotinic acid hydrazide on *Mycobacterium paratuberculosis*. J Am Vet Med Assoc 1953;122:309–10.

6. Gilmour NJL. Studies on the effect of the Rimino Phenazine B633 (G30320) on *Mycobacterium johnei*. Br Vet J 1966;122:517–21.

7. Gilmour NJL. The effect of the Rimino Phenazine B633 (630320) on pre-clinical *Mycobacterium johnei* infection in sheep. Br Vet J 1968;124:492–7.

8. Gilmour NJL, Angus KW. The effect of the Rimino Phenazine B663 (G30320) on *Mycobaterium Johnei* infection and reinfection in sheep. J Comp Pathol 1971;81: 221–6.

9. Slocombe RF. Combined streptomycin-isoniazid rifampine therapy in the treatment of Johne's disease in a goat. Can Vet J 1982;23:160–3.

10. Gilmour NJL. The failure of the Rimino Phenazine B663 (G30320) to reduce the level of experimental *Mycobacterium johnei* infections in calves. Br Vet J 1970;126:5–6.

11. Larsen AB, Kopecky KE. *Mycobacterium paratuberculosis* in reproductive organs and semen of bulls. J Am Vet Med Assoc 1970;31:255–8.

12. Larsen AB, Stalheim OHV, Hughes DE, et al. *Mycobacterium paratuberculosis* in the semen and genital organs of a semen donor bull. J Am Vet Med Assoc 1981;179: 169–71.

13. Kopecky KE, Larsen AB, Merkal RS. Uterine infection in bovine paratuberculosis. Am J Vet Med Assoc 1967;728:1043–5.

14. McQueen DS, Russel EG. Culture of *Mycobacterium paratuberculosis* from bovine fetuses. Aust Vet J 1979;55:203–4.

15. Whittington RJ, Windsor PA. *In utero* infection of cattle with *Mycobacterium avium* subsp. *paratuberculosis*: a critical review and meta-analysis. Vet J 2009;179:60–9.

16. Rhode RF, Shulaw WP. Isolation of *Mycobacterium paratuberculosis* from the uterine flush fluids of cows with clinical paratuberculosis. J Am Vet Med Assoc 1990;197: 1482–3.

17. Sweeney RW. Transmission of paratuberculosis. In: Paratuberculosis (Johne's disease). Vet Clin North Am Food Anim Pract 1996;12:305–12.

18. Physician Desk Reference. 44th edition. Oradell (NJ): Medical Economics; 1990.

19. St-Jean G. Treatment of clinical paratuberuculosis in cattle. Vet Clin North Am Food Anim Pract 1996;12:417–30.

20. Dhillon J, Dickinson JM, Sole K, et al. Preventative therapy of tuberculosis in Cornell model mice with combination of rifampin, isoniazid, and pyrazinamide. Antimicrob Agents Chemother 1996;40:552–5.

21. Somoskovi A, Parsons LM, Salfinger M. The molecular basis of resistance to isoniazid, rifampin, and pyrazinamide in *Mycobacterium tuberculosis*. Respir Res 2001;2: 164–8.

22. Kleeberg H, Worthington RW. A modern approach to the control of bovine paratuberculosis. J S Afr Vet Med Assoc 1963;3:383–90.

23. Kleeberg H, Wixon RC, Worthington RW. Evaluation of isoniazid in the field control of bovine paratuberculosis. J S Afr Vet Med Assoc 1966;37:219–27.

24. Rankin JD. Isoniazid: Its effects on *Mycobacterium johnei* in vitro and its failure to cure clinical Johne's disease in cattle. Vet Rec 1953;65:649–51.

25. Baldwin EW. Isoniazid therapy in two cases of Johne's disease: VM/SAC. Agri Pract 1976;71:1359–62.
26. Dean GS, Rhodes SG, Coad M, et al. Isoniazid treatment of *Mycobacterium bovis* in cattle as a model for human tuberculosis. Tuberculosis 2008;88:586–94.
27. Larsen AB, Vardamam TH. The effect of viomycin, 4:4' diamino diphenyl sulfone, and other agents of *Mycobacterium paratuberculosis*. Am J Vet Res 1952;13:466–8.
28. Smith, BP. Actinomycosis (lumpy jaw). In: Smith BP, editor. Large animal internal medicine. 4th edition. St. Louis (MO): Mosby Elsevier; 2009. p. 784–5.
29. Van Metre DC, Tennant BC, Whitlock RH. Actinomycosis. In: Divers TJ, Peek SF, editors. Rhebun's diseases of dairy cattle. 2nd edition. St. Louis (MO): Mosby Elsevier; 2008. p. 241–4.
30. Mandell GL, Sande MA. Antimicrobial agents, drugs used in chemoherapy of tuberculosis and leprosy. In: Goodman Gilman A, Goodman LS, Rall TW, editors. The pharmacology basis of therapeutics. 7th edition. New York: Macmillan; 1985. p. 1199–218.
31. Hillidge CJ. Use of erythromycin-rifampin combination in treatment of *R. equi* pneumonia. Vet Microbiol 1987;14:337–42.
32. Zanetti S, Molicotti P, Cannas S, et al. "In vitro" activities of antimycobacterial agents against *Mycobacterium avium* subsp. *paratuberculosis* linked to Crohn's disease and paratuberculosis. Ann Clin Microbiol Antimicrob 2006;5:27–30.
33. Krishnan MY, Manning EJ, Collins MT. Effects of interactions of antimicrobial drugs with each other and with 6-mercaptopurine on *in vitro* growth of *Mycobacterium avium* subspecies *paratuberculosis*. J Antimicrob Chemotherap 2009;64:1018–23.
34. Mondal D, Sinha RP, Gupta MK. Effect of combination therapy in *Mycobacterium paratuberculosis* infected rabbits. Ind J Exp Biol 1994;32:318–23.
35. Sweeney RW, Divers TJ, Benson C, et al. Pharmacokinetics of rifampin in calves and adult sheep. J Vet Pharmacol Ther 1988;11:413–6.
36. Jernigan AD, St. Jean G, Rings DM, et al. Rifampin pharmacokinetics in adult sheep. Am J Vet Res 1991;52:1626–9.
37. Pettit JH, Rees RJ. Studies on sulfone resistance in leprosy. 2. Treatment with a rimino phenazine derivative (B.663). Int J Lepr Other Mycobact Dis 1966;34:391–7.
38. Morrison NE, Marley GM. The mode of action of clofazimine DNA binding studies. Int J Lepr Other Mycobact Dis 1976;44:133–4.
39. Eidus L, Denst H. The susceptibility of *Mycobacterium paratuberculosis* (Johne's bacillus) to chemotherapeutic agents. Am Rev Resp Dis 1964;89:289–92.
40. Larsen AB, Vardamam TH. Preliminary studies on the effect of streptomycin and other agents on *Mycobacterium paratuberculosis*. Am J Vet Res 1950;11:374–7.
41. Hintz AM, Merkal RS, Whipple DL, et al. In vivo studies of antimicrobial agents against *Mycobacterium paratuberculosis*. In: Abstracts of the International Colloquium on Research on Paratuberculosis. Ames, IA, National Animal Disease Center, 1983.
42. Chiodini RJ. Bacterial activities of various antimicrobial agents against human and animal isolates of *Mycobacterium paratuberculosis*. Antimicrob Agents Chemother 1990;34:366–7.
43. Greenstein RJ, Su L, Juste RA, et al. On the action of cyclosporine A, rapamycin and tacrolimus on *M. avium* including subspecies *paratuberculosis*. PLoS ONE 2008; 3(6)e2496.
44. Dubuisson T, Bogatcheva E, Krishnan MY, et al. *In vitro* antimicrobial activities of capuramycin analogues against non-tuberculous mycobacteria. J Antimicrob Chemother 2010;65:2590–7.
45. Bogatcheva E, Dubuisson T, Protopopova M, et al. Chemical modification of capuramycins to enhance antibacterial activity. J Antimicrob Chemother 2011;66:578–87.

46. Chiodini RJ. Crohn's disease and the mycobacterioses: a review and comparison of two disease entities. Clin Microbiol Rev 1989;2:90–117.

47. Senturk S, Mecitoglu Z, Ulgen M, Onat K. Effect of levamisole on faecal levels of acid-fast organisms in cows with paratuberculosis. Vet Rec 2009;165:118–9.

48. Gonsette RE, Demonty L, Delmotte P, et al. Modulation of immunity in multiple sclerosis: a double-blind levamisole-placebo controlled study in 85 patients. J Neurol 1982;228:65–72.

49. Szeto CC, Gillespie KM, Mathieson PW. Levamisole induces interleukin-18 and shifts type 1/type 2 cytokine balance in the immune response of experimentally malnourished rats. Immunol 2000;100:217–24.

50. Hili P, Evans CS, Veness RG. Antimicrobial action of essential oils: the effect of dimethylsulphoxide on the activity of cinnamon oil. Lett Appl Microbiol 1997;269-75.

51. Wong SY, Grant IR, Friedman M, Elliott CT, et al. Antibacterial activities of naturally occurring compounds against Mycobacterium avium subsp. paratuberculosis. Appl Environ Microbiol 2008;74:5986–90.

52. Richards WD. In vitro and in vivo inhibition of Mycobacterium paratuberculosis by iron deprivation: A hypothesis. In: Conference on Johne's disease. Australia: 1988, p. 87–94.

53. Click RE, Van Kampen CL. Short Communication: Progression of Johne's disease curtailed by a probiotic. J Dairy Sci 2009;92:4846–51.

54. Click RE, Van Kampen CL. Assessment of Dietzia subsp. C79793-74 for treatment of cattle with evidence of paratuberculosis. Virulence 2010;1:145–55.

55. Larsen AB, Merkal RS, Moon HW. Evaluation of a paratuberculosis vaccine given to calves before infection. Am J Vet Res 1974;35:367–9.

56. Kalis CH, Hesselink JW, Karkema HW, et al. Use of long-term vaccination with a killed vaccine to prevent fecal shedding of Mycobacterium avium subsp paratuberculosis in dairy herds. Am J Vet Res 2001;62:270–4.

57. Sweeney RW, Whitlock RH, Bowersock TL et al. Effect of subcutaneous administration of a killed Mycobacterium avium subsp paratuberculosis vaccine on colonization of tissues following oral exposure to the organism in calves. Am J Vet Res 2009;70: 493–7.

58. Goodrich RD, Garrett JE, Gast DR, et al. Influence of monensin on the performance of cattle. J Anim Sci 1984;58:1484–98.

59. McDougald LR. Monensin for the prevention of coccidiosis in calves. Am J Vet Res 1978;39:1748–9.

60. Duffield TF, Leslie KE, Sandals D, et al. Effect of pre-partum administration of monensin in a controlled-release capsule on milk production and milk components in early lactation. J Dairy Sci 1999;82:272–9.

61. Schelling GT. Monensin mode of action in the rumen. J Anim Sci 1984;58:1518–27.

62. Westley JW, Liu CM, Evan RH Jr, et al. Preparation, properties and biological activity of natural and semisynthetic urethanes of monensin. J Antibiot 1983;36:1195–200.

63. Brumbaugh GW, Frelier PF, Roussel AJ, et al. Prophylactic effect of monensin sodium against experimentally induced paratuberculosis in mice. Am J Vet Res 1992;53: 544–6.

64. Brumbaugh GW, Simpson RB, Edwards JF, et al. Susceptibility of Mycobacterium avium sbsp paratuberculosis to monensin sodium or tilmicosin phosphate in vitro and resulting infectivity in a murine model. Can J Vet Res 2004;68:175–81.

65. Greenstein RJ, Su L, Whitlock RH, et al. Monensin causes dose dependent inhibition of Mycobacterium avium subspecies paratuberculosis in radiometric culture. Gut Path 2009;1:4.

66. Brumbaugh GW, Edwards JF, Roussel AJ, et al. Effect of monensin sodium on histological lesions of naturally occurring bovine paratuberculosis. J Comp Path 2000;123:22–8.
67. Hendrick SH, Duffield TF, Leslie KE, et al. Monensin might protect Ontario, Canada dairy cows from paratuberculosis milk-ELISA positivity. Prev Vet Med 2006;76:237–48.
68. Hendrick SH, Kelton DF, Leslie KE, et al. Efficacy of monensin sodium for the reduction of fecal shedding of *Mycobacterium avium* subsp. paratuberculosis in infected dairy cattle. Prev Med 2006;75:206–20.
69. Whitlock RH, Sweeney RW, Fyock T, et al. Johne's disease: the effect of feeding monensin to reduce the bioburden of *Mycobacterium avium* subspecies *paratuberculosis* in neonatal calves. In: Proceedings of the American Association of Bovine Practitioners Annual Meeting. Salt Lake City, 2005. p. 191–2.
70. Sweeney RW, Whitlock RH, Hamir AN, et al. Isolation of *Mycobacterium paratuberculosis* after oral inoculation of uninfected cattle. Am J Vet Res 1992;53:1312–4.
71. Duffield TF, Bagg RN. Use of ionophores in lactating dairy cattle: A review. Can Vet J 2000;41:388–94.
72. Hall JO. Ionophore use and toxicity in cattle. Vet Clin North Am Food Anim Pract 2000;16:499–505.
73. Potter EL, VanDuyn RL, Coole CO. Monensin toxicity in cattle. J Anim Sci 1984;58: 1499–510.
74. Van Vleet JF, Amstutz HE, Weirich WE, et al. Clinical, clinicopathologic, and pathologic alterations in acute monensin toxicosis in cattle. Am J Vet Res 1983;44:2133–43.
75. Tsan, MF. Mechanism of gallium-67 accumulation in inflammatory lesions. J Nucl Med 1985;26:88–92.
76. Olakanmi O, Britigan BE, Schlesinger LS. Gallium disrupts iron metabolism of mycobacteria residing within human macrophages. Infect Immun 2000;10:5619–627.
77. Harrington JR, Martens RJ, Cohen ND, et al. Antimicrobial activity of gallium against virulent *Rhodococcus equi in vitro* and *in vivo*. J Vet Pharmacol Ther 2006;29:121–7.
78. Kaneko Y, Thoendel M, Olakanmi O, et al. The transition metal gallium disrupts *Pseudomonas aeruginosa* iron metabolism and has antimicrobial and antibiofilm activity. J Clin Invest 2007;117:877–88.
79. Fecteau ME, Fyock TL, McAdams SC, et al. Antimicrobial activity of gallium nitrate against *Mycobacterium avium* subsp *paratuberculosis in vitro*. Am J Vet Res 2011; 72:1243–6.
80. Fecteau ME, Whitlock RH, Fyock TL, et al. Antimicrobial Activity of Gallium Nitrate against *Mycobacterium avium subsp.* paratuberculosis in Neonatal Calves. J Vet Intern Med 2011, in press.

Genetic Susceptibility to Paratuberculosis

Brian W. Kirkpatrick, MS, PhD[a,b,]*, George E. Shook, MS, PhD[b]

KEYWORDS

- Heritability • Gene • Genomic • QTL • WGAS
- Paratuberculosis

Genetics, as an approach to disease control, is an emerging discipline. It can become an adjunct to other disease control approaches such as vaccination, chemotherapy, segregation, and other management practices. Like vaccination and segregation, genetics is a preventive measure. Genetics is a good candidate as a method of preventing infection by *Mycobacterium avium* subsp. *paratuberculosis* (MAP) because currently an effective vaccine is not available and the disease is incurable. Genetic improvement of disease resistance is a slow, long-term process, but the results are permanent; genetic gains made in one generation remain in future generations, and under a program of continuous improvement, advances in genetic resistance accumulate generation upon generation. In contrast, vaccination must be administered to each new individual in each generation. An important role exists for both genetic improvement and vaccination. Research to improve both genetic approaches and vaccines is necessary to advance MAP infection prevention. However, a drawback to vaccination is that it preempts the opportunity to measure genetic susceptibility. And unless a vaccine is highly effective, it also preempts the opportunity to diagnose diseased animals by serology.

The response of an animal to exposure to a pathogen, such as MAP, can be characterized as susceptibility, resistance, or tolerance. Susceptibility is evidenced by infection and progression to a disease state, resistance is characterized by absence of infection or successfully combating an infection and clearing the pathogen, and tolerance is characterized by infection and a muted disease state. Host genetic variation is expected to contribute to varying animal response to pathogen exposure for all these possible exposure outcomes, although in most cases concerning paratuberculosis, the focus of research work has been examination of susceptibility

The authors have nothing to disclose.

[a] Department of Animal Sciences, University of Wisconsin-Madison, 1675 Observatory Drive, Madison, WI 53706, USA

[b] Department of Dairy Science, University of Wisconsin-Madison, 1675 Observatory Drive, Madison, WI 53706, USA

* Corresponding author. Department of Animal Sciences, University of Wisconsin-Madison, 1675 Observatory Drive, Madison, WI 53706.

E-mail address: bwkirkpa@wisc.edu

Vet Clin Food Anim 27 (2011) 559–571
doi:10.1016/j.cvfa.2011.07.003
0749-0720/11/$ – see front matter © 2011 Elsevier Inc. All rights reserved.

vetfood.theclinics.com

to infection. This is in large part a practical matter as resistance or tolerance to infection would be most easily evaluated by a challenge study in which all animals are exposed to an identical pathogen dose and subsequently evaluated over an extended time period. While conceptually straightforward, studies of this type are prohibitively expensive if applied to species such as cattle where individual animal cost is high, disease progression (paratuberculosis) is slow and large numbers of animals are required for genetic analyses. As a consequence, host genetic analyses with cattle have been largely limited to field data and consideration of susceptibility to infection. This chapter reviews the current information regarding genetic variation for suscep- tibility to MAP infection and considers the application of this information in manage- ment of bovine paratuberculosis.

Three kinds of evidence can be used to identify genetic contribution to MAP prevalence: differences among breeds, differences among sire daughter groups, and differences among DNA markers at specific loci. Each will be considered in turn.

BREED DIFFERENCES

In a survey of cattle producers in the United Kingdom,[1] a higher occurrence of Johne's disease was found in herds of Channel Island breed cattle (Jersey, Guernsey) compared to Friesian or other breeds. From the standpoint of study design, a comparison of breeds must be conducted within herds or locations in which the breeds are comingled to ensure comparable MAP exposure. Otherwise, confounding of breed with factors such as geographic location or herd management methods cast doubts that any observed these differences are indicative of breed effects. Regard- less, an examination of 4579 purebred cattle of 14 breeds in Texas found highly significant differences between genetic groups in frequency of positive enzyme-linked immunosorbent assay (ELISA) results.[2] Bos indicus purebreds and crosses (compos- ite breeds) had odds ratios 17-fold and 3.5-fold greater than Bos taurus breeds for positive ELISA results. However, there was concern that seropositive test results may have been due to cross-reactions with some other organism, as several Bos indicus herds showed no other evidence (clinical or microbiological) of Johne's disease. Alternatively, the authors suggested that these results may indicate a successful response of the Bos indicus cattle to MAP infection. A subsequent study[3] also found significantly greater occurrence of seropositive animals with increasing proportion of Bos indicus breeding in a study of 238 cows from an Angus × Brahman diallel cross (sires of both breeds mated to dams of both breeds and F_1 crosses to produce animals of purebred, F_1 and backcross composition). Unlike an earlier study,[2] in this case breed and herd were not confounded as all animals were from a single herd. In a study of sheep breeds,[4] necropsy records from a research population of Romney (n = 2348) and Merino (n = 1297) sheep were used to examine breed differences in incidence of Johne's disease. Incidence was higher in Merino (4.78%) than Romney (3.49%) sheep in that study, a difference that approached statistical significance ($P<.051$). Management of the population was such that sheep of the 2 breeds were comingled on most occasions, except for the times from lambing to docking and single-sire mating. Taken together, these various studies provide evidence of breed or subspecies effects. In contrast, in other studies, such as an epidemiological investi- gation of MAP ELISA, results in culled cattle[5] are informative for differences in infection between classes of cattle (beef vs dairy) but cannot lead to any conclusion concerning breed effects given the confounding of breed and style of animal husbandry. From these studies one can conclude that there is evidence for genetic variability in animal susceptibility to MAP infection and reason to consider genetic improvement for this trait.

Table 1
Heritability estimates for measures of MAP infection in Holstein cattle

References	MAP-Infected Phenotype Definition	No. of Sires	No. of Daughters	Heritability Range
Koets et al[7]	T	586	3020	0.01–0.09
Mortensen et al[8]	ME	NR[a]	11,535	0.091–0.102
Gonda et al[9]	FC, SE, FC, or SE	46	4603	0.091–0.183
Hinger et al[10]	SE	564	4524	0.05–0.13
Attalla et al[11]	ME	NR[a]	21,524	0.065–0.095
Berry et al[12]	SE	816	4789	0.07–0.15

Abbreviations: FC, fecal culture; T, postmortem histology or tissue culture; ME, milk ELISA; SE, serum ELISA.
[a] Not reported.

SIRE LINE DIFFERENCES AND HERITABILITY

A more definitive conclusion can be drawn from studies that examine effects attributable to sire when sires are used across common herds or use similar data in estimation of heritability for MAP infection (**Table 1**). Heritability is the portion of difference between individual animals' phenotypes that is attributable to transmittable genetic effects. Nielsen and colleagues[6] determined the MAP infection status of 7410 Danish dairy cattle on the basis of a milk ELISA. Data from the full data set or a subset comprised of daughter-dam pairs were analyzed for contribution of sire or dam of cow to phenotypic variance (ELISA result). Sire effects accounted for 1.9% and 6.3% of the phenotypic variance, respectively, in the 2 analyses and provided evidence of a genetic component to susceptibility. Several studies[7×11] have estimated heritability for MAP infection using substantial data sets that have included records from 3000 to more than 20,000 cattle. Definition of the MAP-infected phenotype was based on different criteria among these studies, with antibody levels assessed by ELISA being the most common measure. Postmortem analysis of bacterial cultures from intestinal tissue and lymph nodes and histopathology was used to determine infection and disease status in 3020 Dutch dairy cattle in 1 study.[7] Animals testing positive to any of the 3 measures were considered infected for purposes of heritability estimation. Subsequent studies have used ELISA testing of milk[8,11] or blood[10,12] samples to assess infection phenotype. Another study involved a total of 4233 daughters in 12 large sire families used ELISA testing of blood samples in conjunction with fecal testing by culture.[9] Among the 12 sires, predicted apparent prevalence of MAP infection (ie, regressed for number of daughters and adjusted for herd environment) ranged from 5.3% to 10.4%; in other words, in a given herd with moderate to high infection exposure, MAP infection prevalence among daughters of the best bull was half that of the worst bull.[9] Heritability estimates for susceptibility to MAP infection in dairy cattle from these studies ranged from less than 0.01 to 0.18 with most estimates between 0.09 and 0.12 (**Table 1**). Heritability estimates in sheep, although limited to 1 study[4] with 2 sheep breeds, are consistent with those from cattle. Heritability of MAP infection susceptibility was higher in Merino (0.18 ± 0.11) than Romney (0.07 ± 0.14) sheep. In summary, heritability estimates vary within and among studies depending on analytical model and diagnostic tests used to define the infection status of animals (phenotype), but in most cases were significantly different from zero and on the order of approximately 0.10. By way of comparison, these estimates are similar to heritability estimates for somatic cell score (logarithm of somatic cell count) and higher than heritability for clinical mastitis in dairy cattle. This modest heritability indicates that nongenetic management and environmental factors play a large role in causing differences in MAP infection rate among animals; management strategies will always be an important component in control of MAP infection. Nevertheless, useful genetic improvement to reduce MAP infection susceptibility could be possible through progeny testing of sires used for artificial insemination.

Clearly there is evidence for genetic variation in host susceptibility to MAP infection, raising the possibility of genetic improvement programs aimed at reducing the susceptibility to MAP infection of livestock populations. Nonzero estimates of MAP infection susceptibility heritability indicate a genetic contribution to this characteristic but leave unanswered the question of how many and which genes.

DIFFERENCES AMONG DNA MARKERS

Understanding the contribution of specific genes to variation in MAP susceptibility has been the focus of 2 general types of studies, candidate gene studies and whole genome association studies (WGAS). Candidate gene studies reviewed here are examinations of specific genes chosen a priori as candidates based on knowledge of their physiological roles or from knowledge of their association with or causative role in inflammatory bowel diseases in other species. In such studies there is no prior genetic mapping information that associates the candidate gene's genomic region with disease or susceptibility to MAP infection in the species of interest. In contrast, WGAS take a global approach to comprehensively survey the genome of the species of interest for genetic markers (typically single nucleotide polymorphisms [SNPs]) associated with a disease or infection phenotype. A more simple explanation of a SNP is that it is a single base site in the genome of a species where mutation has led to the presence of alternative nucleotides (A, C, G, or T) at that specific site (ie, a polymorphism). Typically, only 2 alternative bases (termed alleles) will be observed—for example, A or C. Consequently, 3 possible genotypes (eg, AA, AC, or CC) are possible considering the alleles inherited by an offspring from mother and father. SNP genotyping then allows one to track the inheritance of a specific chromosomal or genome segment. The particular merit of SNPs as genetic markers is that they are abundant (ie, they occur in literally millions of locations within mammalian genomes), and they are amenable to high throughput genotyping; tens or hundreds of thousands of SNP markers can be simultaneously genotyped on individuals at a cost of a fraction of a cent for each genotype. Results from WGAS provide information that can be used directly in predicting infection susceptibility genetics as well as providing the preliminary information on which *positional* candidate gene studies can be based (identification of a narrow genomic location in which a gene responsible for susceptibility to infection resides). Results from candidate gene studies will be presented first, followed by WGAS, and then a comparison of results.

CANDIDATE GENE STUDIES

Information on which candidate gene studies in ruminants have been based is the current understanding of the role of specific genes governing the immune system or results from analysis of specific genes in model organisms or humans. Concerning the latter, Crohn's disease in humans is an inflammatory bowel disease with manifestations similar to Johne's disease in ruminants. Crohn's disease has been extensively studied genetically, initially through candidate gene and linkage analyses and more recently through WGAS; results from these studies provide some of the candidate

Table 2
Candidate genes associated with susceptibility to *MAP* infection

Gene	Polymorphism	Location (Chromosome/Mb)	References
NOD2 (CARD15)	c.2197 T>C (C733R) c.*1908C>T	18/18.16	Pinedo et al,[14,15] Ruiz-Larranaga et al[16]
TLR1	Val220Met	6/60.36	Mucha et al[17]
TLR2	Ile680Val 1903 T/C	17/4.28	Mucha et al,[17] Koets et al[18]
TLR4	Asp299Asn Gly389Ser	8/112.43	Mucha et al[17]
SLC11A1 (NRAMP)	Microsatellite c.1067C>G (P356A) c.1157–91A>T	2/110.80	Reddacliff et al,[21] Ruiz-Larranaga et al[22]
SP110	c.587A>G (Asp196Ser)	2/122.34	Ruiz-Larranaga et al[31]
IL10RA	633C>A 984G>A 1185C>T	15/27.07	Verschoor et al[19]

Bovine genomic location based on genome assembly Btau4.1

genes considered in ruminant studies of MAP infection. Over 30 genomic regions associated with Crohn's disease have been identified through WGAS and subsequently validated in replication studies or by independent WGAS. In many cases, positional candidate genes (ie, candidates chosen for their proximity to a significant DNA marker in addition to known function) have been evaluated and functionally relevant polymorphisms identified. The human WGAS work is summarized at a National Institutes of Health–supported website (*A Catalog of Published Genome-Wide Association Studies*, http://www.genome.gov/gwastudies/).

Candidate genes for which association with susceptibility to MAP infection in ruminants have been reported are listed in **Table 2**. The first gene listed, nucleotide-binding oligomerization domain containing 2 or *NOD2* (previously referred to as caspase recruitment domain family member 15, or *CARD15*), was one of the first genes identified through genetic studies of Crohn's disease in humans. Multiple deleterious mutations of this gene have been identified in humans with profound effects on predisposition to Crohn's disease.[13] Studies of *NOD2* and Johne's disease in cattle have yielded preliminary associations between *NOD2* polymorphisms and infection status in separate studies with a mixed Angus × Brahman population[14,15] and Holstein-Friesian populations.[16] The associated *NOD2* polymorphisms differed between the 2 studies, which may reflect different functional polymorphisms in the different cattle populations. Unlike the human work, the SNPs associated in these cattle studies are not of obvious direct functional relevance and instead are most likely linked markers for an unknown, functional polymorphism. In both cases, the results should be considered preliminary and requiring replication.

Toll-like receptors 1, 2, and 4 have been reported to have polymorphisms potentially associated with susceptibility to MAP infection in cattle.[17,18] Toll-like receptors are a part of the innate immune system responsible for pathogen recognition and were chosen as candidate genes on this basis. Multiple breeds were used in the initial study,[17] and it is unclear from the report if the contribution of breed was adequately accounted for, leading to concern about the significance of the associations. As in the case of *NOD2*, the more recent study[18] of Toll-like receptor 2 (TLR2) reported association with a different polymorphism than identified in the earlier study. As mentioned previously for *NOD2*, the association of different TLR2 polymorphisms in different studies (different cattle breeds) could reflect different linked functional polymorphisms in different populations. However, as before, significance of these associations is marginal and the results should be considered preliminary.

Interleukin-10 receptor alpha (*IL10RA*) was considered as a candidate gene for bovine susceptibility to MAP infection, along with other members of the interleukin-10 (IL-10) network, based on associations of IL-10 promoter polymorphisms with inflammatory bowel disease in humans.[19] Six synonymous SNPs were identified in *IL10RA* coding regions, and one of these was found to have a significant association with MAP infection after correction for multiple testing (synonymous SNPs are alternative nucleotide triplets that result in the coding of the same amino acid; they produce no change in amino acid sequence of the protein and so are not functionally relevant). The significant SNP was in high linkage disequilibrium with 3 other SNPs, meaning the specific alleles of these 4 SNPs are inherited together as a group in most cases and inheritance at 1 SNP provides the same information as any other. Given the nature of these SNPs it is unlikely that any is directly causal and more likely they represent linked markers.

Susceptibility of mice to infection by several *Mycobacterium* sp. as well as *Salmonella typhimurium* and *Leishmania donovani* has been associated with allelic variants of the solute carrier family 11 member 1 (*SLC11A1*) gene, formerly referred to as the natural resistance-associated macrophage protein 1 (*NRAMP1*) gene.[20] *SLC11A1* functions as part of the innate immune response, helping block bacterial replication as part of the early response to infection. Tentative associations of the *SLC11A1* gene and MHC region with incidence of ovine Johne's disease have been reported[21] based on genotyping of microsatellite markers closely associated with each (microsatellites are typically dinucleotide repeats, eg, . . . CACACACA . . . , that show variation in the number of consecutive repeat units; as a consequence they can be exploited as genetic markers with alleles differentiated based on DNA sequence length). Two flocks of Merino sheep were phenotyped for MAP infections status based on clinical assessment, fecal culture, and necropsy with a total of 106 and 92 ewes used in flocks A and B, respectively. Proportion of ewes positive for paratuberculosis varied from 14% to 71% and 4% to 88%, in flocks A and B, respectively, depending on the criteria used (fecal culture, disease diagnosis, serology, histopathology). Significance levels reported were nominal p-values of <0.05 in most cases, uncorrected for multiple hypothesis testing, implicit in selecting specific microsatellite alleles for comparison. Nonetheless, the most significantly associated alleles were consistent across the 2 flocks, increasing the credibility of the results. Recently a nonsynonymous nucleotide substitution was identified in the bovine *SLC11A1* gene and found to be significantly associated (nominal $P = 2.4 \times 10^{-5}$) in 1 of 2 Holstein-Friesian populations examined.[22] While the association in the second Holstein-Friesian population was nonsignificant after correction for multiple testing (nominal $P > .05$), the same allele was associated with increased susceptibility.

In summary, candidate gene analyses have often been conducted with inadequate statistical rigor, in some cases using thresholds of statistical significance that fall far below those typically used in WGAS. As a result, some of the results reviewed above should be interpreted as preliminary and inconclusive. In the past, candidate gene analyses were often viewed by the investigators as independent studies; however, there has been recognition for some time now that candidate gene analyses should be viewed in the context of multiple significance testing since a series of candidate genes will likely be evaluated for association with the trait of interest.[23]

WHOLE GENOME ASSOCIATION STUDIES

One genome-wide linkage analysis and 4 WGAS for MAP infection or related phenotypes in cattle have been reported, all using commercial dairy cattle of the Holstein breed. Linkage analyses examine the association of alternative alleles inherited from parents in a defined family structure (eg, often paternal half-sib families in cattle), whereas WGAS consider association of alternative alleles at a given genetic marker using animals sampled broadly from the population. The studies vary in definition of MAP infection phenotype and statistical methodology and each will be described in turn. In all WGAS genotyping was performed using the Bovine 50K Bead Chip (Illumina Inc, San Diego, CA), which provides genotype data for 54,001 SNP markers. Slightly different criteria concerning acceptable minor allele frequency and scoring rate (quality control metrics used in SNP data analysis) were used in the various studies, so there are slight differences in the final number of SNPs used between studies; however, the SNPs used in the studies are largely the same and they typically number around 40,000. For purposes of comparing results between studies, all SNP associations exceeding a threshold of $P < 5 \times 10^{-5}$ are listed in **Table 3**.

The first genome-wide analysis for MAP infection in cattle[24] was a linkage analysis considering the contribution of alternative sire alleles. This study used 3 of the largest half-sib families (a total of 1263 daughters) from a larger Holstein resource population composed of 4586 cows sired by 12 different bulls. Infection status was determined by a combination of ELISA and fecal culture testing; animals positive to either test were deemed MAP-infected and animals negative to both tests were considered noninfected. Overall MAP infection prevalence in the three families was 8.5%. The authors conducted the genome-wide scan by first identifying genomic regions of potential interest on the basis of microsatellite genotyping of pooled positive and matching negative samples and testing difference between pools in allele frequency. Genomic regions of interest were then examined more closely by genotyping individuals for additional microsatellites in these regions and performing interval mapping analyses (an analysis that considers the group of markers on a chromosome, rather than considering the markers one-by-one). One chromosomal region on bovine chromosome 20 was found significant at a chromosome-wise $P<.05$. This study lacked power for several reasons including loss of information in estimating allele frequencies from pooled samples, use of only part of the resource population, analysis of only the paternal genetic contribution (within-family linkage analysis) rather than combined effects of linkage and linkage disequilibrium, and sparse marker density.

In the first MAP infection WGAS reported,[25] cows from 3 herds, in New York, Pennsylvania, and Vermont, were used in a case-control design. Phenotypic assessment of infection was based on culture of MAP from tissue or lymph nodes of the small intestine or from feces obtained at necropsy. Animals were classified as tissue-positive if any of the 4 tissue samples yielded MAP detection with the same approach applied to fecal samples. A total of 218 animals were used in the study; 90 animals were classified as tissue-positive and 41 were classified as fecal-positive. Most, but not all, of the fecal-positive animals were also tissue-positive. For analysis of SNP-trait association, a positive phenotype was defined in 4 different ways: tissue-positive (positive for 1 or more tissue samples), shedding (both fecal and tissue-positive), infected (tissue-positive and fecal-negative), and fecal-positive (positive from fecal sample). For shedding and infected phenotypes, the comparison was made with negatives defined as negative to both tissue and fecal tests. For the other

Table 3
SNPs significantly associated with susceptibility[a] to *MAP* infection in WGAS

Chromosome	Location in Mb (References)[b]	Phenotype
1	3.08[25], 17.11[25], 40.76[28], 120.58[26]	T, I, E, To
2	19.39[30], 64.27[26]	M, To
3	111.68[25]	T and I
5	14.42[28], 37.19[28], 73.63[25], 87.14[28], 88.84[28], 106.21[25]	E, E, E, E, T, F
6	51.77[26], 108.23[28]	To, E
7	17.96[28], 19.75[28], 47.69[25], 83.40[28]	E, E, S, E
8	37.26[29], 74.34[25]	F, E
9	0.70[25], 46.36[29]	S and F, E
10	51.10[28], 52.97[28]	E, E
11	30.60[28], 89.70[29]	E, E
12	69.60[29]	E
13	4.74[30], 71.05[30]	M, M
14	53.98[28]	E
15	21.25[26], 69.30[30]	To, M
16	27.19[25]	T
20	31.97[30]	M
21	26.66[25]	T, I
23	48.40[25]	F
25	8.65[30]	M
26	34.88[30]	M
27	45.25[29]	E

[a] Associations nominally significant at $P < 5 \times 10^{-5}$.
[b] Bovine genomic location based on genome assembly Btau4.1.
Abbreviations: E, seropositive; F, fecal; I, tissue positive but fecal negative; M, seropositive and/or fecal positive; S, shedding; T, positive culture from tissue; To, tolerance.

2 positive categories, the control group was all animals not defined as positive for the phenotype. The number of animals in case and control groups under the various phenotypic definitions ranged from 25 to 90 for cases and from 112 to 168 for controls. Sixteen SNPs showed associations exceeding a nominal $P < 5 \times 10^{-5}$ for the various case definitions, though given the proximity of some of the significant SNPs this represents 11 unique loci (**Table 3**). For 3 of these 11, the association was observed for 2 case definitions. The same data were subsequently reanalyzed considering tolerance as the phenotype where tolerance was considered as the degree (quantitative) or presence or absence (case-control analysis) of fecal shedding among animals that were tissue-positive.[26] SNP associations with the tolerance phenotype that exceeded a nominal $P < 5 \times 10^{-5}$ were observed for 4 genomic locations (**Table 3**). A subsequent reanalysis of the same data set suggests an approach for identifying potential candidate genes using data generated from WGAS.[27] In this study, SNP proximity to known genes was determined, following which SNP association with disease status was evaluated, now considering the relative significance of groups of genes that are part of specific mechanistic pathways or cascades. The advantage of this approach is the multiple genes with modest effects that are part of a common pathway may be discernible as a more significant

group, whereas individually their effects might be considered of insufficient significance for further analysis. Results of this initial study were disappointing in that only one significant pathway was observed; however, the approach merits further consideration with larger data sets and higher density SNP data (the latter so that genes can be more effectively considered).

A second WGAS for susceptibility to MAP infection used cows (n = 232) from 6 dairy herds in Ontario with a prior history of a high prevalence of infection.[28] Cases and controls in this study were defined as animals positive (n = 90) or negative (n = 142) to an ELISA for serum antibodies. SNP associations were examined in a 2-stage logistic regression analysis that first considered the effects of the SNPs individually, then in the second stage considered the effects of SNPs nominally significant in the preliminary analysis in the context of a chromosome-by-chromosome analysis accounting for the other SNPs on the chromosome through a principal components approach. A total of 22 SNPs were significantly associated with infection status, representing 13 unique chromosomal regions, after accounting for SNPs in close proximity that likely account for the same locus (**Table 3**).

A third WGAS for susceptibility to MAP infection used cows from 119 herds in the province of Lodi, Italy. Matching case (ELISA positive, n = 483) and control (ELISA negative, n = 483) animals were sampled from the same herd on the same day.[29] Whole genome SNP genotype data were used to account for animal relationship in a mixed-model analysis of SNP associations. Ten SNPs were significantly ($P < 5 \times 10^{-5}$) associated with infection status (**Table 3**) representing 5 or 6 unique chromosomal regions (chromosomal location of 1 significant SNP was unknown. Six of these 10 SNPs were subsequently evaluated on a second group of case and control animals from the same population (n = 277) and 5 of the 6 were significant at a nominal $P < .01$.

A fourth WGAS for susceptibility to MAP infection used 2 resource populations of approximately 5000 cows each, the first including daughters of 12 specific Holstein sires sampled from 300 cooperating herds across the United States and the second including all cows from 6 cooperating herds in Wisconsin.[30] This study used a unique approach of a case-reference rather than the typical case-control design. Given the extensive availability of 50K SNP genotype data from artificial insemination (AI) sires and the availability of pedigree information on the sampled animals, allele frequencies for cases (positive for either blood ELISA or fecal culture) were compared with allele frequencies for AI sires representative of the herd or population in question. Use of this approach enabled maximizing the number of case samples genotyped (n = 521). Data from the 2 resource populations were analyzed both separately and jointly, the latter using a logistic regression approach. Multiple SNP models predictive of susceptibility genetics were developed using a stepwise, logistic regression approach and evaluated for efficacy using cross-validation. The final multiple SNP model included seven SNPs in unique chromosomal locations significant at $P < 5 \times 10^{-5}$ (**Table 3**). The cross-validation analysis indicated that the models developed were only fair predictors (correct prediction of sample rank 73% of the time), with the caveat that the alternative grouping of samples was cases (ELISA and/or fecal positive) versus reference (AI sires reflecting the general population). A comparison of case and control (both ELISA and fecal negative) would likely yield an improved predictive ability.

CURRENT STATUS

Having reviewed these various candidate gene and WGAS reports, the next logical question is how do the results compare? Examination of the genomic locations of associated candidate genes (**Table 2**) and SNPs from WGAS (**Table 3**) provides no indication of commonality in genomic location between candidate gene and WGAS results. Likewise, a comparison of results between WGAS reports indicates no commonality of genomic locations within a reasonable proximity (1 to 2 Mb, maximum). This perplexing result is attributable to several contributing factors. One factor is the sample size used in the studies. The largest studies reported have used approximately 500 case samples, which is roughly equivalent to the smallest human Crohn's disease WGAS and 6-fold smaller than the largest. An increase in sample size would increase statistical power and increase the likelihood of identifying common genomic regions. Another factor is the inherent uncertainty in the phenotypes being evaluated. The MAP culture from tissue samples is probably one of the most reliable phenotypes, but certainly the most difficult to obtain as it requires slaughter of the participating animal. An added problem posed in using this phenotype is the inability to have closely matched case and control samples on the basis of birth date and herd. The ELISA or fecal tests used in most studies are well known to have high specificity but relatively low sensitivity. The result is that cases and controls have greatly different reliability. An animal that has a positive ELISA test or a positive fecal culture results has clearly been exposed to MAP and become infected. In contrast, the animal that has negative results for these tests may be unexposed, truly resistant, or the recipient of a false-negative test result. The use of a combination of ELISA and fecal testing would provide partial improvement in the veracity of a negative (noninfected) classification. Another related factor that may contribute to the lack of concordance of results is a difference in definition of case and a control. There is variation between the reported studies in both the phenotypic data recorded (tissue culture, fecal culture, blood ELISA, milk ELISA) and the interpretation of that data (infected, shedding, tolerant, etc). A whole cascade of events follows an initial exposure to infection. This includes attachment of the pathogen to intestinal lining, crossing through the intestinal wall, recognition of the pathogen, immune response to the pathogen, proliferation of the pathogen, etc. Each step along the way involves different host defense mechanisms and associated genes. Consequently, it should be expected that different diagnostic phenotypes would identify different genes as significantly associated with MAP infection. Not only are there many genes involved in MAP susceptibility, but the genes identified may differ among studies due to the phenotypes used for diagnosis. Finally, to the extent that some of the genetic polymorphisms for MAP susceptibility occur at differing frequency in different cattle populations, it is possible that such loci would be identified in one study but not exist in another. This is probably not a good explanation for the difference in results between the current WGAS studies as all have used Holstein-Friesian cattle. It should be considered though when comparing results from studies using different breeds of cattle.

On a more hopeful note, variation in statistical significance between studies is to be expected, and the summarization of WGAS in **Table 3** is a list of associations truncated by an arbitrary statistical threshold. Were the bar to be lowered, it would be likely that most significant associations reported here would find counterparts in a number of cases in other studies, albeit at a lesser significance level. This is a strong argument for a combined meta-analysis of data from multiple studies. A combined analysis for like phenotypes would lead to a truer picture of genomic regions associated with MAP infection susceptibility.

OUTLOOK

The practical application of this information will be in predicting *genetics* of susceptibility to MAP infection. This is not to be confused with disease status. A positive ELISA result is a biomarker for MAP infection, paratuberculosis. In contrast, a genomic (ie, SNP-based) prediction of infection susceptibility genetics tells the owner which animals are more likely to become infected should exposure occur. Genomic predictions based on the currently available candidate gene data would be of very limited value owing to the lack of validation in most cases and the limited number of loci putatively identified. The WGAS results clearly suggest susceptibility is multigenic or polygenic. Unlike single-gene conditions such as dwarfism in the beef breeds or hair color in Holsteins, genetic susceptibility to MAP infection is caused by many genes. Results from some of the currently reported WGAS suggest the possibility of using multiple SNPs as predictors of genetic merit for infection susceptibility genetics. A meta-analysis of the existing data would no doubt improve predictive ability. This information can be used as the basis for DNA testing aimed at charactering the genetic merit of potential breeding animals for MAP infection susceptibility. In addition to combined or refined analysis of data from the reported field experiments, and its incorporation in commercial DNA tests, it is possible that milk ELISA test results now being more routinely generated may be incorporated in national genetic evaluations. The results may someday be estimates of genetic merit (eg, predicted transmitting abilities) for susceptibility genetics based on hundreds of thousands of phenotypic records. Such genetic evaluations, whether based on DNA markers or large-scale milk ELISA testing, could be used to select bulls in artificial insemination whose progeny are less susceptible to MAP infection.

Using marker information from meta-analysis is the next step in an evolutionary process toward genetic selection against MAP susceptibility. We can expect this to be followed by positional candidate gene analyses at the most promising marker locations. Subsequently, detailed molecular biology studies would establish the specific nucleotide substitutions in each candidate gene that contribute to suscepti-bility. These steps will require large investments and several years. In the meantime, and hopefully in the near future, results from the meta-analysis of the candidate gene and GWAS studies can be implemented to identify sires and dams with decreased susceptibility.

REFERENCES

1. Cetinkaya B, Erdogan HM, Morgan KL. Relationships between the presence of Johne's disease and farm and management factors in dairy cattle in England. Prev Vet Med 1997;32(3-4):253–66.
2. Roussel AJ, Libal MC, Whitlock RL, et al. Prevalence of and risk factors for paratu-berculosis in purebred beef cattle. J Am Vet Med Assoc 2005;226(5):773–8.
3. Elzo MA, Rae DO, Lanhart SE, et al. Factors associated with ELISA scores for paratuberculosis in an Angus-Brahman multibreed herd of beef cattle. J Anim Sci 2006;84(1):41–8.
4. Hickey SM, Morris CA, Dobbie JL, et al. Heritability of Johne's disease and survival data from Romney and Merino sheep. Proc N Z Soc Anim Prod 2003;63:179–82.
5. Pence M, Baldwin C, Black CC 3rd. The seroprevalence of Johne's disease in Georgia beef and dairy cull cattle. J Vet Diagn Invest 2003;15(5):475–7.
6. Nielsen SS, Grohn YT, Quaas RL, et al. Paratuberculosis in dairy cattle: variation of the antibody response in offspring attributable to the dam. J Dairy Sci 2002;85(2): 406–12.
7. Koets AP, Adugna G, Janss LL, et al. Genetic variation of susceptibility to *Mycobac-terium avium* subsp. *paratuberculosis* infection in dairy cattle. J Dairy Sci 2000;83(11): 2702–8.
8. Mortensen H, Nielsen SS, Berg P. Genetic variation and heritability of the antibody response to *Mycobacterium avium* subspecies *paratuberculosis* in Danish Holstein cows. J Dairy Sci 2004;87(7):2108–13.

9. Gonda MG, Chang YM, Shook GE, et al. Genetic variation of *Mycobacterium avium* ssp. *paratuberculosis* infection in US Holsteins. J Dairy Sci 2006;89(5):1804–12.

10. Hinger M, Brandt H, Erhardt G. Heritability estimates for antibody response to *Mycobacterium avium* subspecies *paratuberculosis* in German Holstein cattle. J Dairy Sci 2008;91(8):3237–44.

11. Attalla SA, Seykora AJ, Cole JB, et al. Genetic parameters of milk ELISA scores for Johne's disease. J Dairy Sci 2010;93(4):1729–35.

12. Berry DP, Good M, Mullowney P, et al. Genetic variation in serological response to *Mycobacterium avium* subspecies *paratuberculosis* and its association with performance in Irish Holstein–Friesian dairy cows. Livestock Sci 2010;131:102–7.

13. Hugot JP. CARD15/NOD2 mutations in Crohn's disease. Ann N Y Acad Sci 2006; 1072:9–18.

14. Pinedo PJ, Buergelt CD, Donovan GA, et al. Association between CARD15/NOD2 gene polymorphisms and paratuberculosis infection in cattle. Vet Microbiol 2009; 134(3-4):346–52.

15. Pinedo PJ, Wang C, Li Y, et al. Risk haplotype analysis for bovine paratuberculosis. Mamm Genome 2009;20(2):124–9.

16. Ruiz-Larranaga O, Garrido JM, et al. Genetic association between bovine NOD2 polymorphisms and infection by *Mycobacterium avium* subsp. *paratuberculosis* in Holstein-Friesian cattle. Anim Genet 2010;41(6):652–5.

17. Mucha R, Bhide MR, Chakurkar EB, et al. Toll-like receptors TLR1, TLR2 and TLR4 gene mutations and natural resistance to *Mycobacterium avium* subsp. *paratuberculosis* infection in cattle. Vet Immunol Immunopathol 2009;128(4):381–8.

18. Koets A, Santema W, Mertens H, et al. Susceptibility to paratuberculosis infection in cattle is associated with single nucleotide polymorphisms in Toll-like receptor 2 which modulate immune responses against *Mycobacterium avium* subspecies *paratuberculosis*. Prev Vet Med 2010;93(4):305–15.

19. Verschoor CP, Pant SD, You Q, et al. Polymorphisms in the gene encoding bovine interleukin-10 receptor alpha are associated with *Mycobacterium avium* ssp. *paratuberculosis* infection status. BMC Genet 2010;11:23.

20. Malo D, Vogan K, Vidal S, et al. Haplotype mapping and sequence analysis of the mouse Nramp gene predict susceptibility to infection with intracellular parasites. Genomics. 1994;23(1):51–61.

21. Reddacliff LA, Beh K, McGregor H, et al. A preliminary study of possible genetic influences on the susceptibility of sheep to Johne's disease. Aust Vet J 2005;83(7): 435–41.

22. Ruiz-Larranaga O, Garrido JM, Manzano C, et al. Identification of single nucleotide polymorphisms in the bovine solute carrier family 11 member 1 (SLC11A1) gene and their association with infection by *Mycobacterium avium* subspecies *paratuberculosis*. J Dairy Sci 2010;93(4):1713–21.

23. Lander E, Kruglyak L. Genetic dissection of complex traits: guidelines for interpreting and reporting linkage results. Nat Genet 1995;11(3):241–7.

24. Gonda MG, Kirkpatrick BW, Shook GE, et al. Identification of a QTL on BTA20 affecting susceptibility to *Mycobacterium avium* ssp. *paratuberculosis* infection in US Holsteins. Anim Genet 2007;38(4):389–96.

25. Settles M, Zanella R, McKay SD, et al. A whole genome association analysis identifies loci associated with *Mycobacterium avium* subsp. *paratuberculosis* infection status in US holstein cattle. Anim Genet 2009;40(5):655–62.

26. Zanella R, Settles ML, McKay SD, et al. Identification of loci associated with tolerance to Johne's disease in Holstein cattle. Anim Genet 2011;42(1):28–38.

27. Neibergs HL, Settles ML, Whitlock RH, et al. GSEA-SNP identifies genes associated with Johne's disease in cattle. Mamm Genome 2010;21(7-8):419–25.

28. Pant SD, Schenkel FS, Verschoor CP, et al. A principal component regression based genome wide analysis approach reveals the presence of a novel QTL on BTA7 for MAP resistance in holstein cattle. Genomics 2010;95(3):176–82.

29. Minozzi G, Buggiotti L, Stella A, et al. Genetic loci involved in antibody response to *Mycobacterium avium* ssp. *paratuberculosis* in cattle. PLoS One 2010;5(6):e11117. PMCID: 2886106.

30. Kirkpatrick BW, Shi X, Shook GE, et al. Whole-Genome association analysis of susceptibility to paratuberculosis in holstein cattle. Anim Genet 2011;42(2):149–60.

31. Ruiz-Larranaga O, Garrido JM, Iriondo M, et al. SP110 as a novel susceptibility gene for *Mycobacterium avium* subspecies *paratuberculosis* infection in cattle. J Dairy Sci 2010;93(12):5950–8.

Paratuberculosis Vaccination

Elisabeth A. Patton, DVM, PhD

KEYWORDS

- Johne's • Paratuberculosis • *Mycobacterium* • Ruminants
- Vaccination

Although the earliest record of vaccination for Johne's disease (JD) dates back to 1926, it has not been widely used in the United States.[1] Currently, there is only one approved vaccine for JD in the United States, Mycopar (Boehringer Ingelheim, Ridgefield, CT, USA). It is a whole-cell bacterin consisting of inactivated *Mycobacterium avium* subsp. *paratuberculosis* (also known as MAP) mixed with an oil adjuvant. Although multiple studies on the efficacy of Johne's vaccine have been published, differences in study design and outcome measures have made direct comparisons challenging. The vast majority of such studies, however, have shown a protective effect of vaccination on MAP infection and clinical disease.[2,3]

REQUIREMENTS FOR JOHNE'S DISEASE VACCINATION

Purchase and administration of Johne's vaccine in the United States is limited to veterinarians approved by state animal health officials. Participating states must follow regulations in USDA Veterinary Services Memo No. 553.4, *Mycobacterium Paratuberculosis Bacterin: Use in Johne's Disease Vaccination Programs in Participating States.* The memorandum requires that the herd owner and herd veterinarian enter into an agreement with the state animal health official regarding the use of the vaccine. Several prerequisites must be completed before the agreement can be approved by the state animal health official. These include (1) confirm premises is infected with MAP (ie, at least 1 positive fecal culture or polymerase chain reaction for MAP on individual, pooled, or environmental fecal samples), (2) negative tuberculin test on all test-eligible animals as defined under herd accreditation test in the Bovine Tuberculosis Eradication Uniform Methods and Rules, (3) herd owner and State animal health agency sign agreement for vaccine use. In addition, there are TB testing requirements for purchased replacement stock that must be met prior to introduction of the animals into vaccinating herds.

The author has nothing to disclose.
Wisconsin Department of Agriculture, Trade and Consumer Protection, Division of Animal Health, PO Box 2811, Madison, WI 53708-8911, USA
E-mail address: elisabeth.patton@wi.gov

Vet Clin Food Anim 27 (2011) 573–580
doi:10.1016/j.cvfa.2011.07.004
0749-0720/11/$ – see front matter © 2011 Published by Elsevier Inc.

SPECIFICS OF JOHNE'S DISEASE VACCINE ADMINISTRATION

In the United States, only replacement heifers and bull calves between 1 and 35 days of age are currently eligible to receive JD vaccine. It is administered subcutaneously in the dewlap approximately 1 inch proximal to the brisket. Vaccinated calves must be identified with an official identification, including external identification and a tattoo indicating the animal is a JD vaccinate, in the left ear, as specified by the USDA memorandum on JD vaccine use. A vaccination report must be submitted to the state animal health official by the veterinarian administering the vaccine.

NEGATIVE ASPECTS OF CURRENT JOHNE'S DISEASE VACCINES

There are several disadvantages to the currently available JD vaccines that include risk of granuloma at the injection site, human health risks from accidental inoculation, and interference with diagnostic testing for bovine tuberculosis (TB) and paratuberculosis.

Cattle may develop a granulomatous lesion at the site of JD vaccine injection (**Fig. 1**); however, approximately 80% of lesions are less than 10 cm in diameter and do not appear to cause discomfort.[3] The vaccine is administered in the dewlap region in an effort to prevent trauma to the site, that might exacerbate the granuloma. In rare instances, granulomas may become abscessed and drain.[3] A study using Gudair vaccine (Pfizer, NSW, Australia; not licensed for use in the United States) in sheep showed that 20–25% of vaccinates had a palpable injection site lesion after 12 months of age and no significant losses were noted at slaughter.[4] There is a clinical impression among veterinarians that when using the Mycopar vaccine, fewer vaccination reactions occur when smaller-gauge needles are used (18 gauge or smaller); however, the product is very viscous and must be warmed in order to flow through smaller-gauge needles (personal communication with various Wisconsin veterinarians).

Accidental inoculation of humans with JD vaccines may also cause a granulomatous lesion at the injection site.[5,6] The severity of lesions may depend on the amount of vaccine injected and the amount of trauma to the injection site. In the event of an accidental inoculation, veterinarians are advised to contact their health care provider and state public health office immediately for specific treatment recommendations.

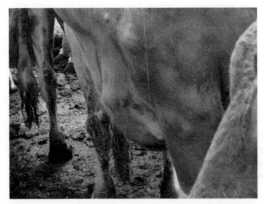

Fig. 1. Granuloma induced by a killed, oil-adjuvanted Johne's disease vaccine. (*Courtesy of* Michael T. Collins, DVM, PhD, Madison, WI.)

Current recommendations for initial treatment include removing the bacterin from the inoculated area by thorough washing and suction. The inoculation site should not be traumatized by squeezing. Reports on treatment of accidental inoculation suggest curettage or excision of the lesion may be the only effective treatment.[6] Other oil-based vaccines have been reported to cause similar lesions.[7] Use of smaller-gauge needles may reduce the amount of trauma and vaccine injected in cases of accidental inoculation. Proper restraint of calves is important to reduce the risk of self-inoculation (**Fig. 2**).

Calves can be vaccinated either in a standing or recumbent position, with care taken to keep the handler's body clear of the area to be vaccinated. The veterinarian administering the vaccine should use a "one-handed" injection technique to reduce the chance of self-inoculation. Care must be taken in disposing of needles after vaccination. Ideally, needles should not be recapped but rather placed directly into a sharps disposal container. Use of shrouded needles has also been suggested as a potential precaution.

Cattle vaccinated with Mycopar develop a cell-mediated response which increases the likelihood of testing positive to the screening test for TB (caudal-fold skin test or CFT). Current bovine TB testing relies on cell mediated immune response to an intradermal injection of *Mycobacterium bovis* purified protein derivative (PPD) antigen. In the US, 2–3% of cattle are expected to have false-positive (FP) test results to the CFT (ie, CFT specificity of 97–98%). Exposure to other mycobacterial organisms can contribute to these FP results. Although results were not statistically significant, a recent study showed that animals testing positive to a MAP ELISA or fecal culture showed a trend toward higher CFT positive rates than in MAP test-negative herd mates.[8] In addition, an increased percentage of JD vaccinated cattle will have higher FP CFT rates as compared to nonvaccinated controls (23% vs 6%, respectively).[3] The effect of JD vaccine on bovine CFT for TB can be prolonged in some animals.[9]

When an animal tests positive to the screening CFT, a confirmatory comparative cervical test (CCT) must be conducted to determine the true infection status of the animal in accordance with federal regulations.[10] The CCT compares the cell-mediated immune response the animal mounts to side-by-side intradermal inoculations of *M bovis* PPD and *M avium* PPD. The CCT for bovine TB can be used as a secondary test to distinguish *M avium* (including MAP) from *M bovis* immune responses. It is performed by state animal health officials and must be completed within 10 days or more than 60 days after the CFT. JD vaccinates typically mount a much larger response to the *M avium* PPD than *M bovis* PPD as determined by skin thickness measurements.[3]

The cost of additional CCT tests in herds with a large number of JD vaccinated animals can become significant for state and federal agencies. Herds with animals testing positive to the CFT are placed under quarantine until the true TB status of the test-positive animal(s) has been resolved. Although herds can still ship milk, animals cannot be moved except under special permit direct to slaughter. These potential costs should be discussed with producers when deciding whether to use JD vaccine as a part of their herd paratuberculosis control program.

In addition to cell mediated responses, JD vaccination induces a humoral immune response in most vaccinated animals, causing animals to test positive on antibody-based diagnostic tests for JD such as ELISA.[9] Because of this, antibody-based JD tests are not reliable to diagnose JD in vaccinated animals. Some JD vaccinating herd owners choose not to test. Those who elect to include MAP testing in their control program have the option of using organism detection-based tests such as fecal culture or fecal polymerase chain reaction as these tests are unaffected by the

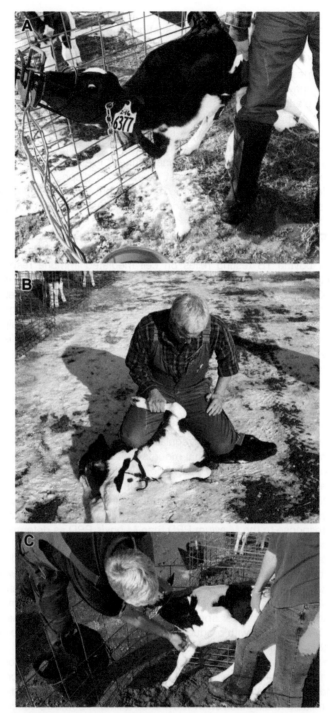

Fig. 2. Safety measures for administration of Johne's disease vaccines. (*A*) Standing calf restraint with a portable headlock. (*B*) Recumbent calf restraint. (*C*) Use of 'one-handed' technique. (*Courtesy of* Jeffery Bohn, DVM, Amery, WI.)

animals JD vaccination status. While the cost of MAP detection-based tests on individual animals are significantly higher than antibody-based tests, fecal sample pooling may be an economical alternative to individual animal testing in some circumstances.[11,12]

EFFICACY OF JOHNE'S DISEASE VACCINATION

JD vaccine does not prevent all new infections; efficacy may depend on age of exposure versus age of vaccination, environmental MAP burden on the farm, and MAP exposure opportunities based on herd management. Most producers and veterinarians that use vaccine find it beneficial in their control program. Further, a majority of studies report that use of the JD vaccine significantly reduces clinical disease, MAP fecal shedding, and MAP tissue burden compared to control animals.[2] It is reasonable to predict that vaccinating herds that integrate best management practices to reduce the risk of MAP transmission, as described in the USDA Johne's disease program standards,[13] will see more significant reduction in disease than will herds using vaccine alone. As with any vaccination program, JD vaccination should be a part of a control program, not the entire program.

WHEN TO USE JOHNE'S DISEASE VACCINE

Restrictions on the use of the JD vaccine in the United States are largely due to the negative aspects of current JD vaccines, as discussed earlier. Many states do not allow JD vaccination and successful JD control has been demonstrated in dairy herds that have not used vaccine.[14] JD vaccine is not necessary for every herd; however, it may help to speed the progress of a JD control program. Indications for JD vaccine are (1) herds with a high MAP infection prevalence (likely to have a heavy environmental MAP burden) or (2) herds that have limited labor, financial, or facility resources and are unable to achieve the management changes needed to reduce the cycle of MAP transmission. Many factors, including cost and benefit of a vaccine program, should be discussed with your client before determining whether vaccine is indicated in a herd's JD control program.

JOHNE'S DISEASE VACCINES IN OTHER COUNTRIES

The use of JD vaccine in Australia's Ovine Johne's Disease Management Plan (OJDMP) is encouraged in all prevalence areas along with pasture and biosecurity planning.[15] The OJDMP is an important part of Australia's National Johne's Disease Control Program (NJDCP). The NJDCP is a program developed with the input of industry and regulatory groups and funded through industry. The OJDMP's 5-year plan was based on aims identified by industry and focuses on reducing risks of purchased animals, use of vaccine, and on-farm best management practices.[15] In 2002, Gudair, a killed JD vaccine, was registered in Australia and is now a central component of their OJDMP. Initial studies using Gudair vaccine demonstrated 90% reduction in clinical JD in sheep, reduced fecal shedding of MAP by 90%, and, in those that did shed, delayed fecal shedding by 1 year compared with nonvaccinated control animals.[4] Additionally, modeling studies demonstrated that heavily MAP-infected flocks, suffering from clinical JD, could expect a return on investment within 2 to 3 years.[16] Gudair vaccine shares some of the same negative aspects as other current JD vaccines, including interference with immunologically based diagnostic tests for paratuberculosis and creation of granulomatous lesions in animals and humans following accidental inoculation.[4,6] Although JD vaccination lesions were found at slaughter in 18% of adult sheep and 65% of lamb carcasses, no economic losses were incurred at slaughter due to these lesions.[17] Gudair is also approved for use in the Australian Goat Johne's Disease Market Assurance Program (GoatMAP) in kids between 4 and 16 weeks of age.[18] Silirum (Pfizer, NSW, Australia),[19] a JD vaccine for cattle, is being evaluated in Australian cattle herds and has recently been shown to reduce fecal shedding and increase milk production compared to nonvaccinating control herds.[20]

NEW VACCINES ON THE HORIZON

Researchers continue to look for new vaccine candidates with improved efficacy and reduced negative side effects.[21] Candidates include subunit vaccines, some of which may have the advantage of not interfering with diagnostic tests for either bovine TB or paratuberculosis. Studies on an HSP70 subunit vaccine demonstrated reduced fecal shedding in an experimental infection model and a lack of interference with current immunodiagnostic assays for bovine tuberculosis and paratuberculosis.[22,23] Injection site lesions using this subunit vaccine were reported to be small with subcutaneous administration and undetectable with intramuscular injection. A JD vaccine without the negative side effects of currently available vaccines would likely require less regulatory oversight and would have the potential to be broadly included in JD control programs.

SUMMARY

Vaccination can be a useful tool in controlling JD. It has been shown to significantly decrease not only clinical disease but also fecal shedding and tissue levels of MAP. However, currently available vaccines have some significant drawbacks that prevent widespread use of JD vaccine in the US JD control program. At present, each state must weigh JD vaccination benefits to herds against the risks of increased costs of bovine TB surveillance and confirmatory testing. In states that allow JD vaccination, practitioners must help herd owners understand and evaluate the costs and benefits of vaccination. MAP infection prevalence, calf exposure rates, and ability to reduce MAP exposure to young stock by improved management are important considerations. In herds where the environmental MAP burden is high or the ability to reduce MAP exposure of young stock through management is limited, the addition of JD vaccine may be important in reducing the cycle of transmission. Ideally, JD vaccine should be used in conjunction with management changes to reduce MAP transmission. Results from Australia's broad use of Gudair vaccine in their sheep JD control program will be highly instructive over the next several years. Research on subunit vaccines appears promising and may provide the MAP infection protection without the negative side effects of current vaccines. Such advances would allow JD vaccination to be broadly incorporated into JD control programs around the globe.

REFERENCES

1. Rosseels V, Huygen K. Vaccination against paratuberculosis. Exp Rev Vaccines 2008;7(6):817–32.
2. Harris NB, Barletta RG. *Mycobacterium avium* subsp. *paratuberculosis* in veterinary medicine. Clin Microbiol Rev 2001;14:489–512.
3. Larsen AB, Moyle AI, Himes EM. Experimental vaccination of cattle against paratuberculosis (Johne's disease) with killed bacterial vaccines: a controlled field study. Am J Vet Res 1978;39:65–9.
4. Reddacliff L, Eppleston J, Windsor P, et al. Efficacy of a killed vaccine for the control of paratuberculosis in Australian sheep flocks. Vet Microbiol 2006;11:577–90.

5. Patterson CJ, LaVenture M, Hurley SS, et al. Accidental self-inoculation with *Mycobacterium paratuberculosis* bacterin (Johne's bacterin) by veterinarians in Wisconsin. J Am Vet Med Assoc 1988;192:1197–9.
6. Windsor PA, Bush R, Links I, et al. Injury caused by self-inoculation with a vaccine of a Freund's complete adjuvant nature (Gudair™) used for control of ovine paratuberculosis. Aust Vet J 2005;83:216–20.
7. O'Neill JK, Richards DM, Ricketts SW, et al. The effects of injection of bovine vaccine into a human digit: a case report. Environ Health 2005;4:21.
8. Dunn JR, Kaneene JB, Grooms DL, et al. Effects of positive results for Mycobacterium avium subsp paratuberculosis as determined by microbial culture of feces or antibody ELISA on results of caudal fold tuberculin test and interferon-gamma assay for tuberculosis in cattle. J Am Vet Med Assoc 2005;226(3):429–35.
9. Muskens J, van Zijderveld F, Eger A, et al. Evaluation of the long-term immune response in cattle after vaccination against paratuberculosis in two Dutch dairy herds. Vet Microbiol 2002;86;269–78.
10. Code of Federal Regulations: 9CFR77 - Tuberculosis. Tuberculosis, 77.1-77.41. 2010. 9. Available at: http://www.gpo.gov/fdsys/search/pagedetails.action;jsessionid=Ns6t NnjDkLRyy8pvSGVGnc1ZRkvyHYCd91tQ2fpC85Y2tGcJpGG1!1866820623! 978953990?browsePath=Title+9%2FChapter+I%2FSubchapter+C%2FPart+ 77&granuleId=CFR-2010-title9-vol1-part77&packageId=CFR-2010-title9-vol1& collapse=true&fromBrowse=true. Accessed August 26, 2011.
11. van Schaik G, Stehman SM, Schukken YH, et al. Pooled fecal culture sampling for *Mycobacterium avium* subsp. *paratuberculosis* at different herd sizes and prevalence. J Vet Diagn Invest 2003;15:233–41.
12. Wells SJ, Godden SM, Lindeman CJ, et al. Evaluation of bacteriologic culture of individual and pooled fecal samples for detection of *Mycobacterium paratuberculosis* in dairy cattle herds. J Am Vet Med Assoc 2003;223:1022–5.
13. USDA-APHIS. Uniform program standards for the voluntary bovine Johne's disease control program (APHIS 91-45-016). 1-40. 9-1-2010. USDA-APHIS. Available at: http://www.aphis.usda.gov/animal_health/animal_diseases/johnes/downloads/johnes-ups.pdf. Accessed August 26, 2011.
14. Collins MT, Eggleston V, Manning EJ. Successful control of Johne's disease in nine dairy herds: results of a six-year field trial. J Dairy Sci 2010;93(4):1638–43.
15. Animal Health Australia. Australia's OJDMP. Available at: http://www.animal healthaustralia.com.au/programs/johnes-disease/ovine-johnes-disease-in-australia/. Accessed August 26, 2011.
16. Bush RD, Windsor PA, Toribio JA, et al. Financial modelling of the potential cost of ovine Johne's disease and the benefit of vaccinating sheep flocks in southern New South Wales. Aust Vet J 2008;86(10):398–403.
17. Eppleston J, Windsor PA. Lesions attributed to vaccination of sheep with GudairГäó for the control of ovine paratuberculosis: post farm economic impacts at slaughter. Aust Vet J 2007;85(4):129–33.
18. Animal Health Australia. GoatMAP. Available at: www.animalhealthaustralia.com.au/aahc/index.cfm?0D72BEBF-E0FD-79AF-8050-F7AE2C273938. Accessed January 24, 2011.
19. Pfizer A. Silirum start up kit. Available at:https://compliance.silirumaustralia.com.au/documents/startup-kit.pdf. Accessed January 24, 2011.
20. Juste R, Alonso-Hearn M, Molina E, et al. Significant reduction in bacterial shedding and improvement in milk production in dairy farms after the use of a new inactivated paratuberculosis vaccine in a field trial. BMC Res Notes 2009;2(1):233.

21. Huygen K, Bull T, Collins DM. Development of new paratuberculosis vaccines. In: Behr MA, Collins DM, editors. Paratuberculosis: Organism, disease, control. Oxfordshire, UK: CAB International; 2010. p. 353–68.

22. Koets A, Hoek A, Langelaar M, et al. Mycobacterial 70-kD heat-shock protein is an effective subunit vaccine against bovine paratuberculosis. Vaccine 2006;24(14): 2550–9.

23. Santema W, Hensen S, Rutten V, et al. Heat shock protein 70 subunit vaccination against bovine paratuberculosis does not interfere with current immunodiagnostic assays for bovine tuberculosis. Vaccine 2009;27(17):2312–9.

Diagnosis of Paratuberculosis

Michael T. Collins, DVM, PhD

KEYWORDS
- Johne's • Paratuberculosis • Diagnosis
- *Mycobacterium avium* subsp. *paratuberculosis*

The emergence of paratuberculosis as a common and costly problem affecting multiple ruminant species led to a surge in research funding internationally, which in turn led to development and validation of multiple diagnostic tests. Today, there are available a greater diversity of accurate and affordable tests for paratuberculosis than for most other ruminant infectious diseases, including brucellosis and tuberculosis, 2 diseases that have been virtually eradicated from most developed countries. There is a suitable diagnostic test for virtually every paratuberculosis testing need. The present-day challenge for practitioners is to select the appropriate test for the intended purpose.

An US expert panel simplified this practitioner dilemma in 2006 by formulating consensus testing recommendations for cattle.[1] **Table 1** is an updated adaptation of those consensus recommendations. This article expands on those recommendations focusing on the most commonly used paratuberculosis diagnostics and nuances of their application and interpretation.

Diagnostic test accuracy and validation are best documented in cattle. Thus, testing recommendations in cattle will be described in most detail and then serve as a model for testing recommendations in other species dealt with at the end.

SEEDSTOCK HERDS

Beef cattle and dairy cattle seedstock herds sell animals for breeding. *Mycobacterium avium* subsp. *paratuberculosis* (MAP)-infected cattle are not suitable as breeding livestock; they will have a shortened herd-life and will likely transmit this incurable, contagious, infectious disease to the buyer's herd. Buyers of breeding livestock (eg, herd replacements) are well advised to request seller assurances that the purchased animals are not MAP-infected. Sellers of breeding livestock should anticipate this request and establish laboratory testing evidence of the MAP-infection status of their herd. If their herd is MAP-infected, they should work aggressively to eradicate the

Disclosure: The author is a paid consultant to IDEXX Laboratories, Inc.
Department of Pathobiological Sciences, School of Veterinary Medicine, University of Wisconsin, 2015 Linden Drive, Madison, WI 53706-1102, USA
E-mail address: mcollin5@wisc.edu

Table 1
Recommended diagnostic tests for cattle by testing purpose

Testing Purpose[a]	Commercial Dairy Cattle	Commercial Beef Cattle	Commercial Goats	Commercial Sheep	All Seedstock
Control program in MAP-infected high prevalence (>5% test-positive) herds	ELISA	ELISA	ELISA	Pooled fecal culture or PCR	Fecal culture or PCR on individual animals
Surveillance	Environmental or pooled fecal culture	Confirmatory testing of clinical suspects	Environmental or pooled fecal culture	Environmental or pooled fecal culture	NR
Eradication	Pooled fecal culture or pooled fecal PCR	Pooled fecal culture or pooled fecal PCR	Pooled fecal culture or pooled fecal PCR	Pooled fecal PCR	Fecal culture or PCR on individual animals
Confirm a clinical diagnosis on animals in herds with no prior confirmed MAP infections	Necropsy, fecal culture, or PCR on the affected individual	Necropsy, fecal culture, or PCR on the affected individual	Necropsy, fecal culture, or PCR on the affected individual	Necropsy or fecal PCR on the affected individual	Culture or PCR and histopathology on biopsy or necropsy-collected tissues
Confirm a clinical diagnosis on animals in herds proved to be MAP infected	ELISA, fecal culture, or PCR	ELISA, fecal culture, or PCR	ELISA, fecal culture, or PCR	Fecal PCR	Culture or PCR and histopathology on biopsy or necropsy tissues

NR = not recommended; seedstock herds should either be classified as test-negative (Table 2) or work toward this goal.

[a] Other purposes not listed: herd classification (see Table 2); biosecurity (see Fig. 1).

Data from Collins MT, Gardner IA, Garry FB, et al. Consensus recommendations on diagnostic testing for the detection of paratuberculosis in cattle in the United States. J Am Vet Med Assoc 2006;229(12):1912–9.

infection (see elsewhere in this issue for paratuberculosis control in beef and dairy herds). Practitioners should recommend the best testing program to serve their client's interests, whether a livestock buyer or seller. Obviously, they should avoid the conflict of interest that occurs by advising both the seller and buyer.

There are official rules regulating classification herds of low MAP infection risk in many countries and practitioners must be familiar with the latest rules for their region. **Table 2** provides the testing requirements of the US Voluntary Bovine Johne's Disease Control Program (VBJDCP).[2] Seeking official (eg, governmental) recognition of the MAP herd status is the best advice for clients selling breeding livestock. In the absence of an official MAP herd status, prepurchase testing can help prospective cattle buyers limit their risk of buying MAP-infected cattle. Risk management through testing is outlined as a decision tree in **Fig. 1**.[1]

Seedstock herd owners are commonly reluctant to test for paratuberculosis, fearing that a positive diagnosis will damage their reputation. It is the practitioner's challenge to explain that the herd's reputation will be damaged more if a customer discovers they bought an MAP-infected animal than by getting confidential MAP test results on a herd and disclosing those results, when requested, to help their customers purchase non–MAP-infected animals.

As described elsewhere in this issue, multiple herd-level prevalence surveys demonstrate that the odds favor the likelihood that any given US beef herd is not MAP-infected. Therefore, beef cattle herd owners can expect "good news" from a herd screening test. A screening test is rapid and low cost but not necessarily 100% specific. A positive screening test, such as by enzyme-linked immunosorbent assay (ELISA) for antibodies in serum or milk, is not proof positive that the tested animal is MAP-infected. Only if a confirmatory test, based on detection of MAP by culture or polymerase chain reaction (PCR), is definitive evidence the tested animal, and thus the herd, is MAP-infected.

Analogies to screening tests for cancer may help clients understand the value of testing their herd. Screening humans for colon, prostate, or breast cancer is not fun and people justifiably fear positive results. However, these tests are widely recommended because early detection leads to early and more successful treatment. Not doing such screening tests may result in discovering diseases in their late, more advanced, and sometimes untreatable stages. Screening tests on humans are always followed by more specific confirmatory tests. The same holds true for paratuberculosis in many situations.

Seedstock buyers should request to see the most recent MAP herd test and should buy only MAP test–negative cattle from test-negative dams in low or zero MAP test prevalence herds. Seedstock sellers should conduct annual whole-herd tests in compliance with official herd classification programs or testing regimens of comparable rigor. The guidelines in the US Program Standards (**Table 2**) offer epidemiologically sound testing strategies and interpretation criteria, based on herd size, thereby simplifying practitioner testing recommendations to seedstock producers. When judging the merits of a customized, nonofficial, herd testing program, look for testing regimens that test a large proportion of the adult herd on a random basis using well-recognized, validated, laboratory assays (commercial kits preferred) performed by NVSL-approved laboratories. The more years-worth of test data following a consistent testing regimen, the greater is the knowledge of the true MAP-infection status of the herd.

MAP is an obligate pathogen, unable to replicate outside its animal host. While persistent in the environment, it slowly dies off after leaving its host. Therefore, eradication of paratuberculosis from a herd or flock is theoretically possible, although proof this can be accomplished has not been published. Eradication of MAP from a population requires both good herd management and the most sensitive diagnostic tests, fecal culture or PCR. Animals

Table 2
Herd testing strategies to achieve JD herd classification levels

Herd Size	Testing Strategy	Herd Classification Level					
		1	2	3	4	5	6
1–99		Maximum proportion positive to achieve level (no rounding)					
	ELISA	≤1.5%	0%				
	ELISA+ Individual MAPDT		0%				
	Individual MAPDT	≤6.0%	≤2.0%	0%	0%	0%	0%
	Pooled MAPDT	≤15.0%	0%	0%		0%	0%
	Environmental MAPDT	0%					
100–199	ELISA	≤2.5%	≤1.5%	≤0.5%	0%	0%	0%
	ELISA+ Individual MAPDT	≤1.0%	0%				
	Individual MAPDT	≤6.5%	≤3.5%	≤1.5%	0%	0%	0%
	Pooled MAPDT	≤15.0%	≤10.0%	0%		0%	0%
	Environmental MAPDT	0%					
200–299	ELISA	≤3.5%	≤2.0%	≤1.0%	0%	0%	0%
	ELISA+ Individual MAPDT	≤1.5%	≤0.5%	0%			
	Individual MAPDT	≤7.0%	≤4.0%	≤1.5%	0%	0%	0%
	Pooled MAPDT	≤13.0%	≤10.0%	≤6.0%	0%	0%	0%
	Environmental MAPDT	0%					
≥300	ELISA	≤4.0%	≤2.5%	≤1.0%	0%	0%	0%
	ELISA+ Individual MAPDT	≤2.0%	≤1.0%	≤0.5%	0%	0%	0%
	Individual MAPDT	≤7.5%	≤5.0%	≤2.0%	0%	0%	0%
	Pooled MAPDT	≤11.0%	≤7.0%	≤5.0%	0%	0%	0%
	Environmental MAPDT	0%					

Herd size = No. test-eligible animals (ie, all female cattle ≥36 mo old and male cattle ≥24 mo Old). The minimum number of cattle to test for each herd size is listed in the Program Standards.
MAPDT = MAP direct detection test (eg, based on culture or PCR).
ELISA + Individual MAPDT = ELISA on individuals animals with follow-up individual MAPDT on ELISA-positives.
Environment MAPDT is only available for dairy herds; not beef herds.
Shaded cells indicate that this testing option is not available. It is for statistical reasons that pooled MAPDT is not allowed to reach level 4 for herds of <200 test-eligible cattle; yes, it seems counterintuitive.
For additional explanatory details, see: Available at: http://www.aphis.usda.gov/animal_health/animal_diseases/johnes/downloads/johnes-ups.pdf. Accessed August 23, 2011.
Adapted from USDA-APHIS. Uniform Program Standards for the Voluntary Bovine Johne's Disease Control Program. 1–40. 9-1-2010. Fort Collins (CO): USDA-APHIS. APHIS 91-45-016. Available at http://www.aphis.usda.gov/animal_health/animal_diseases/johnes/downloads/johnes-ups.pdf. Accessed August 23, 2011.

Johne's Disease Biosecurity for Beef and Dairy Seedstock Herds

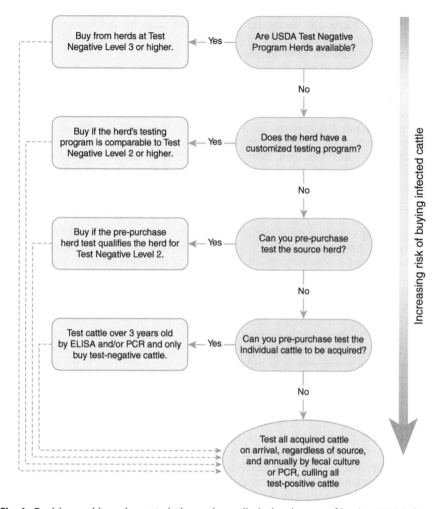

Fig. 1. Decision making scheme to help producers limit the chances of buying MAP-infected cattle. "Test Negative level" refers to herd classification criteria established by the US Voluntary National Bovine Johne's Disease Control Program. (*Adapted from* Collins MT, Gardner IA, Garry FB, et al. Consensus recommendations on diagnostic testing for the detection of paratuberculosis in cattle in the United States. J Am Vet Med Assoc 2006;229(12): 1912–9; with permission.)

found positive must be removed from the herd or flock promptly. Efforts must span multiple years, even well beyond the first whole-herd negative test.

COMMERCIAL BEEF CATTLE HERDS

Paratuberculosis surveys around the globe repeatedly have found that MAP-infections are more common in dairy than beef cattle herds (see Epidemiology article by

Lombard elsewhere in this issue). The herd-level paratuberculosis prevalence estimate for commercial cow-calf (suckler) beef cattle in the United States is less than 8%.[3] Some experts think that registered seedstock herds have a higher infection rate than commercial cow-calf herds, but this has not been proved by surveys using diagnostic tests. Therefore, practitioners can approach beef cattle herds with the presumption they are not MAP-infected.

Commercial cow-calf operations have limited economic motivation to determine if their herd is MAP-infected or to implement control programs involving testing, a clear-cut out-of-pocket expense. Modeling experts in the United Kingdom disagree with this viewpoint.[4] It remains to be seen if their model can be validated with field data. Thus, unless the owners of a commercial cow-calf operations perceives paratuberculosis to be a concern for his/her herd and requests testing, it seems pointless to try and convince them to test for MAP based only on economic considerations. If they do wish to test, they can follow the recommendations for beef cattle seedstock herds described earlier.

COMMERCIAL DAIRY HERDS

Commercial diary herds in most regions of the world have a high probability of being MAP-infected, based on published herd-level prevalence data.[5,6] Consequently, practitioners should work to definitively determine the MAP-infection status of all commercial dairy herds in their practice—a form of triage to focus MAP control efforts on the herds most needing it. This can be done in a variety of ways, the best being by necropsy of one or more cattle clinically suspected to have paratuberculosis (ie, with diarrhea or unexplained weight loss in the face of a normal appetite). If a field necropsy is performed, thickened portions of intestinal and enlarged gastrointestinal tract–associated lymph nodes should be submitted to a diagnostic laboratory fresh and formalinized for microbiology and histopathology, respectively. In the absence of grossly visible pathology, the following 4 tissues should be collected at a minimum: ileum, lower jejunum, and ileocecal and mesenteric lymph nodes.

Two alternatives to necropsy for herd-level confirmation of MAP-infection are (1) fecal culture or PCR on 30 cattle culled from the herd for poor production ("targeted testing") and (2) culture or PCR of environmental fecal samples from at least 6 sites on the farm where cattle comingle.[7–9] Testing targeted at cattle being culled helps assess the degree to which paratuberculosis is forcing involuntary culling decisions, a parameter that producers can roughly translate to the economic impact of the disease in their herd. The number of MAP-positive environmental fecal cultures is loosely related to the within-herd infection prevalence.[9,10]

Commercial dairy herds found not to be MAP-infected should consider heightened efforts to (1) prove the herd is not infected (ie, as for seedstock herds described earlier) and (2) remain not infected by completely closing the herd or by imposing stringent testing requirements on cattle entering the herd, just as for seedstock producers.

MAP-infected commercial dairy herds must gauge the economic impact of the infection and develop an appropriate level of response (ie, improved herd management to limit MAP-infection transmission supported by regular testing to find and manage or cull the infectious cows). This often begins with a herd risk assessment. Details of paratuberculosis control in dairy herds are described elsewhere in this issue. From a diagnostic testing perspective, it is important to note that low-cost, indirect tests for paratuberculosis, based on antibody detection in serum, plasma, or milk samples, provide accurate and affordable tools to effectively support paratuberculosis control programs, as proved in field studies.[11–14] Such tests are most often done using ELISA technology, and several commercial ELISA kits for paratuberculosis are available globally.

Use of ELISAs is most appropriate in herds meeting the following 2 criteria:

1. The herd has been confirmed MAP-infected by an organism detection–based test (ie, culture or PCR).
2. The approximate within-herd apparent (ELISA) prevalence of paratuberculosis is greater than 5%. At lower within-herd prevalences, more specific tests such as culture or PCR are required in order to have sufficiently high predictive value to warrant actions based on test results; pooling samples helps contain the cost of culture or PCR testing.

When ELISAs are used to support paratuberculosis control in dairy herds, 3 principles must be observed:

1. Heifer rearing management practices to limit infection transmission must first be identified and implemented; it is useless to use paratuberculosis tests on a herdwide basis unless herd management is first fixed.
2. ELISA results should be interpreted quantitatively (ie, positive results should be graded as low, medium or high [strong] positive). All ELISAs produce quantitative results and laboratories have the option to provide that data in addition to results interpretations to clients.[15]
3. Actions based on the magnitude of ELISA result should be prescribed *before* initiation of the testing program and should be strictly adhered to, regardless of the clinical status of the animals.

An example of ELISA interpretation and actions, based on diagnostic predictive values and economic decision analysis, is outlined in **Table 3**.

Large commercial dairy herds tend to have a low and steady-state paratuberculosis prevalence, commonly less than 5%. Management practices on these dairies are typically good at keeping the infection from spreading. However, these herds commonly buy untested cattle from herds of unknown MAP-infection status and thus routinely introduce MAP-infected herd replacements. In the United States, roughly 5% to 10% of these random source cattle will be MAP-infected and detectable by ELISA (see information on animal-level prevalence in the Epidemiology article by Lombard elsewhere in this issue). These cattle will produce less milk than expected and be culled from the herd prematurely, resulting in an economic loss equal to most of the purchase price of each affected animal.[16] Prepurchase testing strategies to limit this loss are strongly advised. A simple strategy is to stipulate in contracts with cattle dealers the delivery of only ELISA-negative cattle. Any premium paid for cattle meeting this standard will likely be more than offset by losses resulting from purchase of ELSA-positive (probably MAP-infected) dairy replacements.

GOATS

Diagnostic tests for paratuberculosis in goats are comparable in accuracy to those in cattle and the same principles and recommendations generally apply. The cost advantage of ELISAs makes then particularly useful to support control programs. Because cross-reactivity can occur with the common disease caseous lymphadenitis (CLA), caused by *Corynebacterium pseudotuberculosis*, practitioners are advised to check with the testing laboratory to ensure the ELISA kit used is suitable for paratuberculosis diagnosis in goats. Reports indicate that the 2 currently available commercial ELISA kits in the United States—Parachek (Prionics AG, Zurich,

Table 3
ELISA interpretation and action plan for confirmed MAP-infected commercial dairy herds with a moderate to high (eg, >5% test prevalence)

ELISA Result	Interpretation	Recommended Actions
Negative	High probability of **not** being MAP-infected, depending on overall within herd prevalence.	The cow is probably not infectious even if MAP infected. She is safe for use as a colostrum donor and safe for calving in group maternity pens.
Low-positive	Moderate probability of MAP infection. Occasionally animals will revert to test-negative on the next lactation.	Keep the cow for one additional lactation unless clinical signs of paratuberculosis develop. If allowed to calve, limit all opportunities for MAP infection transmission to calves.
Medium-positive	High (>85%) likelihood of MAP infection but may not become clinically affected during the current lactation.	Consider culling the cow if any other health or production problems occur. If allowed to calve, limit all opportunities for MAP infection transmission to calves.
High-positive	Very high (>98%) probability of MAP infection and shedding of MAP in feces.	Do not breed this cow. Cull the cow for slaughter at the end of her lactation. This cow is highly infectious; a major source of MAP on the farm.

Switzerland) and HerdCheck (IDEXX-Pourquier, Westbrook, ME, USA)—do not cross-react with CLA.[17,18] Goats comingled with MAP-infected sheep may acquire the sheep strain of MAP, making diagnosis by culture more difficult, owing to its fastidious growth requirements. However, in the United States, the sheep strain of MAP has yet to be identified in goats without a history of being exposed to sheep. When such a history exists, producers should be encouraged to use PCR testing in place of culture.

SHEEP

Serologic tests are less useful in sheep than in goats. Multiple studies have shown that while ELISAs have improved over the past 2 decades, they identify a different subset of sheep than the AGID test, with only about a 50% to 60% overlap.[19,20] This causes difficulty as even clinically affected sheep can be negative on one test and positive on the other. Unless sheep have been exposed to MAP-infected cattle, goats, or deer, sheep in the United States are usually infected with sheep strains of MAP. Sheep strains are very difficult to culture, and even culture systems optimized for growing sheep strains are less sensitive than for the detection of cattle strains. Therefore, PCR is the most effective currently available test for MAP diagnosis in sheep. The higher cost of PCR compared to ELISA can be managed by pooling of fecal samples, but the pooling strategy should be designed to fit the goals of the producer. Australian researchers have shown that most infected flocks can be identified by pooling fecal samples from 50 sheep. However, this method is only valid if 6 to 7 pools of feces from individual adult sheep are tested and at least 2% of the ewes have the multibacillary form of paratuberculosis.[21,22] This type of surveillance is not appropriate in smaller US flocks. If producers would like to identify as many shedding sheep as possible but would like to pool fecal samples to reduce costs, following the cattle guidelines of 5 animals per fecal pool is a reasonable approach. While not yet experimentally verified, PCR testing of environmental fecal samples, as is recommended for dairy cattle, may be one of the most cost-effective ways to survey a flock's MAP-infection status.[7] This is easily accomplished when freshly sheared ewes are kept in dry lots just prior to lambing.

OTHER RUMINANTS

MAP detection tests such as culture and PCR are the most reliable methods for paratuberculosis diagnosis in ruminants where serologic response to MAP-infections have not been well characterized, making the accuracy of serodiagnostic tests unknown.

THE FUTURE

Tests for cellular immunity, such as the skin test for tuberculosis, are notably absent from this article. Such tests are the backbone of tuberculosis control programs and considerable research efforts have been expended to develop such tests for paratuberculosis. Prospects for such assays are limited for 3 reasons: (1) MAP-specific antigens that universally stimulate cytokines or other indicators of cellular immunity in all MAP-infected animals have yet to be discovered, (2) it is unclear if animals with a strong cellular immune response are succumbing to or controlling the infection, and (3) such assays are inherently expensive. Thus, even if such assays were available, it is unclear if or how they would be used. The cost of diagnostics is a major factor in paratuberculosis control programs; the control program must not exceed the cost of the disease.[23] The economics of testing will only change if MAP is considered a zoonotic agent and society decides to mandate, and share the cost of, paratuberculosis control programs on farms. For vaccination to become a viable paratuberculosis control tool, low-cost diagnostic methods to distinguish MAP-vaccinates from animals with MAP-infections must be co-developed with the vaccine.

SUMMARY

The majority of US commercial dairy herds are MAP-infected and should invest in cost-effective control programs that combine herd management changes with a testing program designed to identify the most infections cattle in the herd. Once a commercial dairy herd is confirmed infected by culture or PCR, ELISAs used on serum, plasma, or milk offer the most affordable tests to support control programs. These ELISAs should be used quantitatively and linked to culling or management decisions based on the magnitude of the ELISA result—level of antibody in the clinical sample. Seedstock producers should seek official recognition for having an MAP test-negative herd. If infected, seedstock producers should work to eradicate MAP from their herds using culture or PCR on individual animals with or without first pooling samples. Commercial cow-calf beef cattle producers may not have a sufficiently strong economic incentive to invest in MAP control efforts. Testing of goats generally follows dairy cattle testing recommendations, but for sheep, PCR remains the single most effective diagnostic test. The high cost of PCR testing can be mitigated by using sample pooling.

REFERENCES

1. Collins MT, Gardner IA, Garry FB, et al. Consensus recommendations on diagnostic testing for the detection of paratuberculosis in cattle in the United States. J Am Vet Med Assoc 2006;229(12):1912–9.
2. USDA-APHIS. Uniform Program Standards for the Voluntary Bovine Johne's Disease Control Program. 1–40. 9-1-2010. Fort Collins (CO): USDA-APHIS. APHIS 91-45-016.
3. Dargatz DA, Byrum BA, Hennager SG, et al. Prevalence of antibodies against *Mycobacterium avium* subsp *paratuberculosis* among beef cow-calf herds. J Am Vet Med Assoc 2001;219:497–501.
4. Bennett R, McClement I, McFarlane I. An economic decision support tool for simulating paratuberculosis control strategies in a UK suckler beef herd. Prev Vet Med 2010;93:286–93.
5. Nielsen SS, Toft N. A review of prevalences of paratuberculosis in farmed animals in Europe. Prev Vet Med 2009;88(1):1–14.
6. USDA-APHIS-VS-CEAH. Johne's disease on U.S. dairies, 1991-2007. N521.0408, 1-4. 4-1-2008. Fort Collins (CO): USDA-APHIS-VS-CEAH.
7. Aly SS, Anderson RJ, Whitlock RH, et al. Reliability of environmental sampling to quantify *Mycobacterium avium* subspecies *paratuberculosis* on California free-stall dairies. J Dairy Sci 2009;92(8):3634–42.
8. Kalis CHJ, Hesselink JW, Barkema HW, et al. Culture of strategically pooled bovine fecal samples as a method to screen herds for paratuberculosis. J Vet Diagn Invest 2000;12(6):547–51.
9. Wells SJ, Godden SM, Lindeman CJ, et al. Evaluation of bacteriologic culture of individual and pooled fecal samples for detection of *Mycobacterium paratuberculosis* in dairy cattle herds. J Am Vet Med Assoc 2003;223:1022–5.
10. van Schaik G, Pradenas F, Mella N, et al. Diagnostic validity and costs of pooled fecal samples and individual blood or fecal samples to determine the cow- and herd-status for *Mycobacterium avium* subsp. *paratuberculosis*. Prev Vet Med 2007;82(1–2):159–65.
11. Collins MT, Eggleston V, Manning EJ. Successful control of Johne's disease in nine dairy herds: results of a six-year field trial. J Dairy Sci 2010;93(4):1638–43.
12. Kudahl AB, Nielsen SS, Ostergaard S. Economy, efficacy, and feasibility of a risk-based control program against paratuberculosis. J Dairy Sci 2008;91(12):4599–609.
13. Nielsen SS, Krogh MA, Enevoldsen C. Time to the occurrence of a decline in milk production in cows with various paratuberculosis antibody profiles. J Dairy Sci 2009;92(1):149–55.
14. Nielsen SS. Use of diagnostics for risk-based control of paratuberculosis in dairy herds. In Practice 2009;31:150–4.
15. Collins MT, Wells SJ, Petrini KR, et al. Evaluation of five antibody detection tests for bovine paratuberculosis. Clin Diagn Lab Immunol 2005;12:685–92.
16. Lombard JE, Garry FB, McCluskey BJ, et al. Risk of removal and effects on milk production associated with paratuberculosis status in dairy cows. J Am Vet Med Assoc 2005;227(12):1975–81.
17. Gumber S, Eamens G, Whittington RJ. Evaluation of a Pourquier ELISA kit in relation to agar gel immunodiffusion (AGID) test for assessment of the humoral immune response in sheep and goats with and without *Mycobacterium paratuberculosis* infection. Vet Microbiol 2006;115(91):101.

18. Whittington RJ, Eamens GJ, Cousins DV. Specificity of absorbed ELISA and agar gel immuno-diffusion tests for paratuberculosis in goats with observations about use of these tests in infected goats. Aust Vet J 2003;81(1–2):71–5.
19. Hope AF, Kluver PF, Jones SL, et al. Sensitivity and specificity of two serological tests for the detection of ovine paratuberculosis. Aust Vet J 2000;78(12):850–6.
20. Robbe-Austerman S, Gardner IA, Thomsen BV, et al. Sensitivity and specificity of the agar-gel-immunodiffusion test, ELISA, and the skin test for detection of paratuberculosis in United States Midwest sheep populations. Vet Res 2006;37:553–64.
21. Dhand NK, Sergeant E, Toribio JA, et al. Estimation of sensitivity and flock-sensitivity of pooled faecal culture for *Mycobacterium avium* subsp. *paratuberculosis* in sheep. Prev Vet Med 2010;95(3-4):248–57.
22. Whittington RJ, Fell S, Walker D, et al. Use of pooled fecal culture for sensitive and economic detection of *Mycobacterium avium* subsp *paratuberculosis* infection in flocks of sheep. J Clin Microbiol 2000;38(7):2550–6.
23. Dorshorst NC, Collins MT, Lombard JE. Decision analysis model for paratuberculosis control in commercial dairy herds. Prev Vet Med 2006;75:92–122.

Control of Paratuberculosis in Beef Cattle

Allen J. Roussel, DVM, MS

KEYWORDS

• Paratuberculosis • Cattle • Control • Beef

PREVALENCE

Worldwide, paratuberculosis is less prevalent in beef cattle than in dairy cattle. For this reason, paratuberculosis is considered by some to be a "dairy cattle" disease. While the prevalence of paratuberculosis is less in beef cattle than in dairy cattle, paratuberculosis nevertheless occurs in beef cattle and is a major health and production problem in some herds. Awareness of paratuberculosis among beef cattle producers is generally lower than it is among dairy cattle producers. A study conducted by the National Animal Health Monitoring System (NAHMS) and published in 1997 revealed that nearly 70% of beef producers said they had never heard of paratuberculosis, while a similar study a year earlier showed that only 10% of dairy cattle producers had not heard of the disease.[1,2] Compared to studies of dairy cattle, studies of the prevalence of paratuberculosis of beef cattle are much fewer in number. In the NAHMS study of beef cattle herds in the United States which used the serum enzyme-linked immunosorbent assay (ELISA), only 0.4% of animals had a positive test results.[1] This compares with 2.5% of dairy cattle in a similar study 1 year previously.[2] Among beef herds, 7.9% of herds had at least 1 positive test.[1] This compares to 21.8% of dairy herds.[2] The testing strategy used in this study was designed to identify herds with a prevalence of 10% or greater. In the author's experience, the prevalence in most extensively reared beef cattle herds is less than 10%. Therefore, the true herd prevalence may have been underestimated in this study. Several smaller and less statistically valid surveys of beef cattle in the United States have been published in the past 20 years. Among these studies, the animal-level seroprevalence of paratuberculosis ranged from 3% to 9.6%, while the herd prevalence based on 1 or more seropositive animals ranged from 34% to 76%.[3–6] There are several biases and potential sources of error in the studies, as most of the herds were self-selected and the seroprevalence was not corrected for test sensitivity and specificity. However, the studies suggest that paratuberculosis does in fact affect a substantial number of beef cattle in the United States. Two

The author has nothing to disclose.

Department of Large Animal Clinical Sciences, Texas A&M University, 4475 TAMU, College Station, TX 77843-4475, USA

E-mail address: Aroussel@cvm.tamu.edu

doi:10.1016/j.cvfa.2011.07.005
vetfood.theclinics.com

Canadian studies reported an animal prevalence of 0.8% and 1.5% and a herd prevalence of 15.2% and 28.5% for beef cattle.[7,8]

ECONOMIC IMPACT

The economic impact of paratuberculosis on beef cattle has not been accurately estimated. The low within-herd prevalence, along with the paucity of complete records for many beef herds, makes determining the economic impact of paratuberculosis in beef cattle challenging. Losses associated with death, the sale of underweight cattle, and the replacement costs associated with the disease are obvious. It could reasonably be assumed that a decrease in milk production occurs in beef cattle as it does in dairy cattle; therefore, the weight of calves produced by *Mycobacterium avium* subsp. *paratuberculosis* (MAP)–infected cows would likely be lighter. Other less obvious costs might include the potential loss of sales by purebred producers, the cost of litigation, the cost of the loss of very valuable genetic material, the loss of export markets and the loss of consumer confidence. Most of these costs are hidden or opportunity cost, not out-of-pocket losses. Therefore, the motivation to invest in control programs is low for many beef cattle producers. In fact, for most commercial beef cattle producers with low prevalence herds, there is little economic advantage in investing in paratuberculosis control as long as MAP is considered solely an animal pathogen.

CONTROL STRATEGIES

Two simple goals are foundational for the control of paratuberculosis in any infected herd of cattle, regardless of type: (1) minimize or eliminate the exposure of susceptible calves to the feces of infected cattle and (2) reduce the environmental contamination by eliminating animals that shed MAP. For uninfected herds, the only control measure needed is biosecurity: do not allow infected cattle to enter the property. These principles are so elegantly simple to articulate and so very difficult to execute consistently due to technological and logistical challenges and the resistance of many producers to accept stringent biosecurity practices.

Control strategies available for beef cattle compared to dairy cattle are different. In order to try to understand the differences, it is important to consider the possible reasons why they exist. Obvious differences between beef and dairy cattle in most parts of the developed world include breed, environmental conditions, feeding practices, and calf-rearing practices. While there is no solid evidence that beef breeds are more, or less, susceptible than dairy breeds, there appear to be differences among beef breeds, at least when serologic prevalence is used as an estimate for MAP infection rate. A higher seroprevalence in Brahman compared to Angus cattle was reported within a moderately sized herd.[9] Also, among crossbred cattle within the herd, the seroprevalence was positively correlated with the percentage of Brahman in the pedigree. There is substantial evidence of genetic variability to susceptibility to *Mycobacteria* among cattle. Therefore, it stands to reason that breed differences as well as individual genetic differences might exist. In purebred cattle in Texas, a greater seroprevalence was found in *Bos indicus* and *Bos indicus*–influence herds compared to *Bos taurus* herds.[6] In all of these studies, seropositivity based on a serum ELISA was used to define prevalence. There was evidence of cross-reactivity from environmental mycobacteria in some of the *Bos indicus* herds in the studies.[10] A possible alternative explanation of the high seroprevalence observed is that *Bos indicus* cattle may be more seroreactive to mycobacterial antigens whether they be MAP or other soil-borne *Mycobacteria*. A recent study has identified certain loci associated with seroreactivity to MAP in Holstein cattle.[11] This may explain differences in seroprevalence.

The environmental conditions under which most beef cattle are reared differ from those of dairy cattle. It should be noted that the environment of intensively reared beef cattle that are housed in winter, calved in sheds or barns, and held in close confinement may resemble dairy cattle more than it does that of extensively reared beef cattle. Here, the term "beef cattle" should be considered to mean extensively reared beef cattle. Extensively reared beef cow calf herds are fed stored forage less and are grazed more than the majority of dairy cattle in North America. Perhaps the most important difference between beef cattle and dairy cattle when considering the transmission and control of paratuberculosis involves calf-rearing practices. Almost all calves on modern dairies are separated from their dams within 24 hours of birth. Beef calves typically remain with their dams for 6 to 7 months. Consequently, the exposure of beef calves to the manure of mature cattle is much greater on most beef cattle operations than on most dairy cattle operations.

Cognizant of the differences between beef cattle and dairy cattle, we will now explore control practices aimed at reducing the transmission of paratuberculosis among beef cattle. Based on the biology of the organism, the pathogenesis of the disease, and observational and experimental data derived from dairy cattle, it is possible to suggest a number of control measures that *should* be effective at reducing the transmission of paratuberculosis among beef cattle. Regrettably, there is very little hard evidence that these methods are effective. We are left, therefore, with recommendations that make biological sense but are unproved and cannot be evaluated for cost-effectiveness.

Nursing Calves

Any control program for paratuberculosis in cattle should begin with calves, as they are the most susceptible sector of the population. The potential for control of paratuberculosis in beef herds is limited by the fact that separation of calves from mature cows is not practical. However, any practices that reduce the exposure of calves to the feces of cows is likely to help reduce the transmission of paratuberculosis. Reducing the exposure of calves to the feces of cows can be accomplished using strategies that reduce environmental contamination as well as contamination of feed and water sources. Specifically, the area where calves are born and nursed for the first few months of life can be enlarged. It is important to remember that the "effective" area, not the actual size of the pasture, is the key factor. For example, cattle that have access to a section of land, but have feed, water, and shelter in one corner of the pasture, do not effectively use the entire section. Both environmental contamination and feed contamination can be influenced by the manner in which hay is fed. Most experts now agree that hay from large bales is most effectively used when spread on the ground in amounts that can be consumed in a day or so. Hay rings tend to aggregate cattle and produce muddy areas around the ring during times of precipitation. This leads to mud and fecal contamination of the teats and udder. Researchers have found MAP on the udders of a high proportion of nonshedding beef cows infected in herds where poor sanitation practices were employed. Feeding hay on the side of a hill and moving the feeding area daily is more effective in reducing fecal contamination. Feeding more hay than cattle can consume in 24 hours leads to the transition of hay as feed to hay that cows lie on (eg, hay as bedding). When calves lie down on and perhaps nibble on leftover hay that has been contaminated with the feces of mature cattle, the risk of fecal-oral transmission of pathogens increases. It is known that MAP can survive for many months in pond water. Therefore, pond water could be a source of infection, especially for young calves during their more susceptible period. In a study of risk factors for paratuberculosis in beef cattle, having running streams as a water source reduced the risk of seropositivity in the herd.[6]

Postweaning

After weaning, beef calves are still susceptible to infection with MAP, although less so than are young calves. Weaned calves should be housed or pastured in areas free of the feces of mature cattle. Water and feed sources should also be free of fecal contamination. Because it is now known that some calves shed MAP before reaching maturity, in heavily infected herds the risk of calf-to-calf transmission should be minimized by avoiding overcrowding and optimizing sanitation practices. Ideally, young cattle should remain separated from the mature herd for as long as possible.

While mature cattle are the most resistant to infection with MAP, this resistance can be overcome by massive exposure. Therefore, in heavily infected herds, sanitation practices that reduce fecal contamination to food and water sources of mature cattle should be adopted. These practices should already have been in place for the cow-calf pairs and should be kept in place in the cow herd after weaning.

Segregation and Culling

An obvious strategy to help control transmission in beef herds is to immediately cull all clinical cases. Too often, a thin cow is placed in the corral, dewormed, and fed supplemental feed in an attempt to "put some weight on her." Treatment sometimes leads to an extended stay on the ranch or farm while the slaughter withdrawal time is being observed. Frequently, the corral in which the sick cow is placed is the same corral used to hold weak and sick calves just after calving. In infected herds, any cattle with early signs of possible Johne's disease (weight loss and diarrhea) should be isolated and tested or culled immediately. The isolation area (sick pen) should not be an area used to hold calves. It is frequently recommended that the last calf from any cow that develops clinical Johne's disease should be culled. This recommendation is logical because transmission of paratuberculosis can occur in utero, through colostrum, through milk, and via the fecal-oral route, and the calf is in close contact with its dam during its most susceptible period in life. It stands to reason that the risk of dam-to-calf transmission should be much higher in a beef herd than in a dairy herd because beef calves remain with their dams longer. In 1 study, when herd of origin was not considered, a beef calf from a serologically positive cow was more likely to be serologically positive than was a calf from a serologically negative cow.[12] However, when the herd of origin was factored in the statistical model in a similar study, a calf born to a seropositive dam was not at higher risk of being seropositive than was a calf from a seronegative dam.[13] The findings in these studies suggest that the question of culling calves from infected cows is up for debate. At this time, however, it seems reasonable to cull the last calf from a clinically affected cow with Johne's disease. This recommendation may gain additional credence as we learn more about the genetic susceptibility and resistance to paratuberculosis. Another recommended strategy for control of paratuberculosis in beef herds is to cull thin cows. Because thin beef cows are typically not reproductively efficient and tend not to wean heavy calves, there are other good reasons to cull them in addition to paratuberculosis.

The value of test-and-cull programs in dairy herds, compared to control programs without testing, has been debated for years. Testing and culling are probably more important in beef herds than in dairy herds. Infected cows cannot be separated from calves, and therefore retaining them in the herd increases the potential for contamination of the environment and transmission of infection. In some situations it may be feasible to maintain 2 herds: 1 herd of test-positive cattle and 1 herd of test-negative cattle. The wisdom of this practice may depend upon the test used and the interpretation of this test to make decisions for segregation. All cattle that are fecal culture-positive are shedding MAP in feces, at least at the time of testing. Many cattle with a high positive ELISA result also are shedding. However, a smaller proportion of cattle with moderate and low positive ELISA results are shedding MAP due to the biology of the disease and the fact that at lower ELISA values, false-positive ELISAs are more frequent. Therefore, creating a herd of ELISA suspect, low-positive, and moderate-positive cows makes more sense than a herd of ELISA strong-positive or fecal culture-positive cows. Strong ELISA-positive and fecal culture-positive cattle can be collected for germ plasma (semen and embryos) with little risk of transmission to the offspring.

BIOSECURITY

Producers with infected herds should make every effort to keep their herds uninfected. Very few beef cattle are marketed with information about the paratuberculosis status of the animal or the herd. If information is not provided, buyers should ask sellers about the paratuberculosis status of their herd. Ideally, animals should be purchased only from very low-risk, test-negative herds participating in an official paratuberculosis control program. These herds, however, are not numerous. In some situations, in some areas and in some breeds, it is probably better to purchase cattle from a known infected herd with a good control program, good records, and a low prevalence than from a herd in which the paratuberculosis status is unknown or, perhaps more appropriately stated, "undisclosed." For a more complete discussion on testing strategies, refer to the Diagnosis. Beef cattle producers should be particularly cautious when purchasing embryo transfer recipients and nurse cattle. These are frequently dairy or dairy cross animals. Because the prevalence of paratuberculosis is greater in dairy cattle, the risk of introducing the disease into a beef herd is greater when these cattle are added to the herd. Another potential break in biosecurity is the acquisition of colostrum, especially from dairy herds. High-quality, safe, and effective commercial dry colostrum substitutes are now available, obviating the need for frozen colostrum from other farms. The Voluntary Bovine Johne's Disease Control Program managed by USDA-APHIS was established in the 1990s to help producers control paratuberculosis in their herds. An excellent risk assessment tool is available online at http://www.aphis.usda.gov/animal_health/animal_diseases/johnes/downloads/johnes-umr.pdf.

REFERENCES

1. Dargatz DA, Byrum BA, Hennager SG, et al. Prevalence of antibodies against *Mycobacterium avium* among beef cow-calf herds. J Am Vet Med Assoc 2001;219(4): 497–501.
2. Wells SJ, Wagner BA. Herd-level risk factors for infection with *Mycobacterium paratuberculosis* in US dairies and association between familiarity of the herd manager with the disease or prior diagnosis of the disease in that herd and use of preventive measures. J Am Vet Med Assoc 2000;216(9):1450–7.
3. Merkal RS, Whipple DL, Sacks JM, et al. Prevalence of *Mycobacterium paratuberculosis* in ileocecal lymph nodes of cattle culled in the United States. J Am Vet Med Assoc 1987;190(6):676–80.

4. Keller LL, Harrell CD, Loerzel SM, et al. Johne's disease: seroprevalence of *Mycobacterium avium* subspecies *paratuberculosis* in Florida beef and dairy cattle. Bovine Pract 2004;38(2):135–41.
5. Pence M, Baldwin C, Black CCIII. The seroprevalence of Johne's disease in Georgia beef and dairy cull cattle. J Vet Diagn Invest 2003;15:475–7.
6. Roussel AJ, Libal MC, Whitlock RL, et al. Prevalence of and risk factors for paratuberculosis in purebred beef cattle. J Am Vet Med Assoc 2005;226(5):773–8.
7. Scott HM, Sorensen O, Wu JT, et al. Seroprevalence of and agroecological risk factors for *Mycobacterium avium* subspecies *paratuberculosis* and *neospora caninum* infection among adult beef cattle in cow-calf herds in Alberta, Canada. Can Vet J 2007;48(4):397–406.
8. Waldner CL, Cunningham GL, Janzen ED, et al. Survey of *Mycobacterium avium* subspecies *paratuberculosis* serological status in beef herds on community pastures in Saskatchewan. Can Vet J 2002;43(7):542–6.
9. Elzo MA, Rae DO, Lanhart SE, et al. Factors associated with ELISA scores for paratuberculosis in an Angus-Brahman multibreed herd of beef cattle. J Anim Sci 2006;84(1):41–8.
10. Roussel AJ, Fosgate GT, Manning EJB, et al. Association of fecal shedding of mycobacteria with high ELISA-determined seroprevalence for paratuberculosis in beef herds. J Am Vet Med Assoc 2007;230(6):890–5.
11. Minozzi G, Buggiotti L, Stella A, et al. Genetic loci involved in antibody response to *Mycobacterium avium* ssp. *paratuberculosis* in cattle. PLoS One 2010;15(6):e11117.
12. Osterstock JB, Fosgate GT, Cohen ND, et al. Familial associations with paratuberculosis ELISA results in Texas longhorn cattle. Vet Microb 2008;129:131–8.
13. Osterstock JB, Fosgate GT, Cohen ND, et al. Familial and herd-level associations with paratuberculosis enzyme-linked immunosorbent assay status in beef cattle. J Anim Sci 2008;86:1977–83.

Control of Paratuberculosis in Dairy Herds

Franklyn Garry, DVM, MS, ACVIM

KEYWORDS

- Johne's • Paratuberculosis • Dairy cattle • Control
- Prevention

The basic principles of Johne's disease (JD) control on dairies are relatively straightforward. This contagious, infectious disease, caused by *Mycobacterium avium* subsp. *paratuberculosis* (MAP), is primarily spread via fecal-oral transmission. Because infected animals disseminate the organism through multiple organ systems, spread can also occur in utero and via milk and colostrum. Therefore, these routes of infection require a good control program. Efforts to decrease the within-herd MAP infection prevalence involve 3 basic steps: (1) prevent exposure of susceptible animals to the infectious agent, with particular emphasis on the most susceptible animals; (2) identify and eliminate MAP-infected animals from the herd; and (3) prevent entry of infected animals into the herd. Although there are numerous means to accomplish these 3 steps, there is value in recognizing how straightforward these principles really are and communicating this effectively to producers.

JD has become a very important dairy cattle disease in the United States. It is an insidious disease that can be easily introduced into a herd, and its prevalence gradually increases unless control programs are effectively used. The disease has substantial negative effects on cow productivity and thus can have a major financial impact on a herd.[1,2] The infectious agent is likely a zoonotic pathogen, and humans may be exposed via a variety of routes, with the primary source being MAP-infected animals on dairies. Recent studies have shown that the majority of dairies in the United States have infected animals.[3] For all of these reasons, it is important that dairy veterinarians work with dairy producers to establish effective JD control programs.

There are 2 aspects to JD control programs that will be reviewed here. First is the *strategy* that underlies development of an effective control program, and second is the consideration of *specific control points* in the program that deserve special emphasis.

The author has nothing to disclose.
Department of Clinical Sciences, Integrated Livestock Management, Colorado State University, 300 West Drake Road, Fort Collins, CO 80523, USA
E-mail address: fgarry@colostate.edu

Vet Clin Food Anim 27 (2011) 599–607
doi:10.1016/j.cvfa.2011.07.006
0749-0720/11/$ – see front matter © 2011 Elsevier Inc. All rights reserved.

STRATEGY FOR DEVELOPING A JOHNE'S DISEASE CONTROL PROGRAM

The complications and impediments to establishing an effective control program for JD on dairies arise less from the nature of the disease and more from some historical and current realities about modern dairy production and economics, veterinary involvement with dairy disease control programs, and recognition of the importance of this infectious disease to dairy animal well-being. Until the late 1990s, most veterinarians assumed this disease was not common and was relatively unimportant to the dairy industry. Therefore, the disease was not commonly monitored and veterinarians did not educate producers about the problem. Most dairy producers were unfamiliar with the disease.[3] Dairy producers are highly focused on keeping costs of production low and tend to focus on animal health issues from an economic cost point of view. The possibility that MAP could infect humans has not historically been considered likely, and even now there is no general consensus that this is a zoonotic pathogen.[4] Until the late 1990s, there was no well-defined national disease control program for this problem. Even now, the national program remains voluntary.[7]

Because of these features, most dairy cattle veterinarians have not been involved in JD control efforts until recently. Because JD control remains voluntary, most dairy producers only take action if they believe the problem is economically important for their operation. Because there is no general acceptance that MAP represents a threat to human health, dairy manufacturers do not pay premiums for milk from JD test–negative herds and there is limited government financial aid to assist control efforts. Tuberculosis and brucellosis control programs have been mandated and historically well-funded by the federal government, so program implementation targeted at those diseases requires little discussion with producers. By contrast, development of a voluntary, biosecurity-based control program for JD, where there is no highly effective vaccine and there is no treatment, presents an uncommon veterinary challenge. For practitioners who are looking to establish JD control programs on dairies, mastitis control programs may provide a good general model to follow. Most other dairy cattle infectious disease control programs have typically relied primarily on vaccination and disease treatment. For all of these reasons it is important to discuss the strategy behind establishment of a biosecurity-based, voluntary JD control program as well as the practical aspects of JD control.

ELEMENTS OF A JOHN'S DISEASE CONTROL PROGRAM STRATEGY

The National Voluntary Bovine Johne's Disease Control Program (VBJDCP) was established in 1998.[5] This program proscribes 3 essential elements that should be conducted in sequence: (1) education, (2) developing a risk assessment and management plan, and (3) developing a testing program.

Producer Education

Any voluntary dairy management or disease control program requires that the owner or dairy manager make decisions. These range from decisions about whether to institute a control program at all, to decisions about purchasing animals, investing time and effort to change management practices and facility design, to decisions about testing strategies and animal treatment or culling. Creating a good control program therefore requires that the owner or manager is well-informed and has a sound knowledge base on which to make these decisions. For the herd veterinarian, taking time to ensure that the producer is well-informed not only facilitates decision-making but also reinforces the trust and respect that are required for a good veterinarian–producer relationship.

Historically, US dairy producers have been very poorly informed about JD. The nationwide educational initiatives that have taken place over the past decade have had a dramatic impact in helping producers understand the nature and the importance of this disease problem. The knowledge required to develop and maintain a robust control program goes beyond the level of general information. Educational materials have been developed and are available from multiple sources, including the state Johne's disease coordinator, the U.S. Animal Health Association, and online sources (**Table 1**).

Before a control program is established, it is important that the producer understands the nature of JD and how it spreads in a herd. Producers should be informed about the various aspects of a good JD control program and why certain steps in the program are higher priority than others. It is also important for a producer to understand the benefits of a well-managed JD control program for dairy herd health and profitability. The benefits, liabilities, and costs of various testing strategies should be discussed. Although some producers will choose to take no further action to control JD on the dairy, the herd veterinarian should continue to update producers as new JD information becomes available. Many producers will choose to take the next step and pursue the development of a JD risk assessment and management plan.

The educational process should include a discussion of the difference between "cost" and "investment". For many dairy producers, any financial outlay is seen as a cost, and most producers strive to attain the lowest possible cost of production. Control of JD requires inputs of both time and money. A control program should have definable objectives and these objectives must have a value to the producer. For the JD control program to work, it is important to establish the long-term goals to determine if the costs of the program will be wise investments for long-term profitability. It is particularly helpful to consider the benefits of a control program not just in the context of decreasing JD prevalence but also in terms of other benefits that may accrue, such as improved maternity pen management leading to improved calf health. These features of the control program are often not considered in the benefit-cost investment equation if the focus of discussion centers exclusively on JD losses.

RISK ASSESSMENTS AND MANAGEMENT PLANS

Materials have been developed to serve as a template for conducting JD risk assessments and developing JD management plans for dairies.[6] These materials include an instructional guide and a handbook. The standardized forms provided in the handbook are designed to help establish a common understanding of the producer's overall goals for the operation, the health challenges faced by the operation, the producer's priority on JD control compared to other farm concerns, the major risks for MAP transmission, and a prioritized list of steps the producer can take to decrease spread of the disease.

Collecting this information and establishing a management plan will usually take a couple hours of on-farm time but is arguably the most important step in establishing a control program to which the producer will adhere. Because the instructional guide is very thorough, the details of this process will not be repeated here. The goal of performing a risk assessment and management plan (RAMP) is to develop a practical and affordable control program that the producer understands and to which the producer is committed. There are several aspects of this process that are worth emphasizing.

Evaluating the goals of the operation is important to determine how high a priority to place on JD control. For a seedstock producer, for example, maintaining access to

Table 1
Online sources of information about Johne's disease and control programs targeted at both veterinarians and producers

Resource	URL
Johne's Information Center	http://johnes.org/
Johne's Information Central	http://johnesdisease.org/
USDA-APHIS Johne's Disease Information	http://www.aphis.usda.gov/animal_health/animal_diseases/johnes/index.shtml
Johne's Disease Veterinary Certificate Program	http://vetmedce.vetmed.wisc.edu/jdvcp/
Animal Health Australia	http://www.animalhealthaustralia.com.au/programs/jd/jd_home.cfm
Danish Control Program on Bovine Paratuberculosis	http://www.landbrugsinfo.dk/Kvaeg/Sundhed-og-dyrevelfaerd/Paratuberkulose/Sider/Op_Paratb_UK.aspx

markets for the animals will be different than maintaining access to the milk market for a commercial producer. For producers facing very significant challenges with other disease problems, JD control may appropriately be a lower priority. Alternatively, some other disease challenges may require exactly the same steps as those entailed in a JD control program, such that a JD program can provide benefit beyond simply reducing the prevalence of JD. Establishing how much emphasis to put in the JD control program should therefore be a very important discussion between the practitioner and the producer.

Properly conducted, the general information component of the RAMP enhances the herd veterinarian's understanding of the whole operation (i.e., the "big picture"). This step should help integrate the JD control program into an overall herd health management plan.

Involving the producer in the risk assessment is important. Confronted with the challenge of determining where disease transmission risks occur on the dairy, most producers will be more motivated to institute changes in herd management than if they are provided with a list established independently by the herd veterinarian. All JD control programs are unique to the individual dairy because of the large variation between dairies in producer goals, focus on other dairy challenges, priority assigned to JD, and other features of dairy herd management.

Once the risks for MAP transmission have been agreed upon by the producer and herd veterinarian, the management plan is constructed. For most dairies, there will be numerous opportunities to decrease spread of disease from cows to calves. Constructing a good management plan that will actually be implemented on the dairy requires that the various potential control opportunities are prioritized. For most dairy operations, this prioritization is critically important and only the top few management changes should be implemented at one time to avoid making the task overwhelming. The complexity of dairy herd management and aspects of human nature dictate that trying to implement too many changes at once often results in no individual change actually being implemented well.

The management plan should be built with clearly defined objectives that are both short-term and long-term goals. These objectives should be measurable and realistic. The management plan should be practical and integrate with other aspects of overall herd health. The plan must be constructed with the active participation of the producer, which underscores the importance of effective producer education prior to this step.

TESTING PLANS FOR JOHNE'S DISEASE CONTROL

The tests available to determine MAP infection status have different costs, different characteristics, and different turnaround times.[7] Therefore, certain tests are better suited for particular purposes and these are well described in the Diagnostics article by Collins elsewhere in this issue.

Some testing will commonly have been done prior to the development of a management plan, and this will be helpful in establishing whether MAP infection is present on the dairy and a crude estimate of infection prevalence. Establishing an ongoing testing plan, however, should usually be the last step in developing a JD control program. The value of testing depends heavily on the purpose of the testing and what it will accomplish. Testing will often represent the single biggest ongoing cash outlay for JD control and therefore must be justified based on how the results will be used in the management plan.

Testing costs are an investment in the JD control strategy and should be used to identify cows in the herd that are most infectious. If test results are used to identify cows whose colostrum or milk will not be fed to calves or to identify cows that will be kept out of the maternity area or whose calves will not be kept as heifer replacements, then the return on investment in testing costs is generally well justified.[8] For some management plans, however, testing may not be included. Other producers may want to document that the herd is free of MAP infection, requiring extensive herd testing using the most sensitive tests.[9] The important point is that the testing plan should be constructed for to achieve a specific purpose.[7]

CONTROL POINTS FOR A JOHNE'S DISEASE PROGRAM

Having considered fundamental strategies, the JD control program itself may be viewed as analogous to the Hazard Analysis Critical Control Points (HACCP) process, now used as the backbone of the US food safety system.[10] The hazards for transmission of MAP to susceptible animals have been identified and our understanding of these hazards is refined through research that evaluates MAP transmission risks via fecal, colostrum and milk contamination, and likelihood of transmission in utero (see Epidemiology article by Lombard elsewhere in this issue). These transmission risks should be conveyed to producers as part of the education program. The on-farm risk assessment evaluates the control points where action can be taken to decrease MAP transmission risk. During this process the producer and veterinarian discuss, and hopefully agree, about whether critical limits for those control points have been exceeded. The action plan is then predicated on mitigating those risks. The plan is documented and actions are implemented (i.e., become standard operating procedures or written protocols on the farm). Periodically thereafter, typically at yearly intervals, but perhaps more frequently for specific activities, the implementation is monitored and recorded.

Much like an HACCP plan, there is no single risk mitigation step that will assure complete JD control (ie, no failsafe step). Therefore, management plans need to implement "multiple hurdles," each of which diminishes the potential for MAP infection transmission to susceptible animals. This is an important concept in the management plan and should be reiterated as the plan is reviewed. Reducing MAP infection prevalence in a herd is a long-term project, and each program review should ensure that the previous steps have been instituted and new refinements and additional hurdles to MAP transmission considered.

It was mentioned earlier that the management plan should include a limited number of management changes at any time, and then should only include new management procedures when the earlier steps have been instituted and become routine. Another useful concept to share with dairy producers is that the chosen management changes should start with those assigned highest priority (ie, of most importance in MAP transmission). Assigning priority for management changes to combat JD should be based on the expected cost-benefit, considering likely impact of the change on JD transmission and other herd health objectives, plus ease and cost of implementation.

PRIORITIZING JOHNE'S DISEASE CONTROL PROCEDURES

The risk assessment process included in the national program, and detailed in the dairy handbook, lists over 30 specific assessment questions. The number of points assigned to each of these questions is designed to reflect expert opinion on the highest priority areas—areas where MAP transmission is most likely to occur. Maternity pen management and preweaned heifer rearing practices are the highest priority areas for JD control on dairies. Baby calves are the individuals most susceptible to new infection on a dairy. Furthermore, steps taken to improve maternity pen management, improve colostrum management, decrease fecal exposure of newborn calves, and improve milk hygiene all decrease risk of other calfhood diseases and therefore leverage JD control processes to improve overall calf health and performance. Some of these steps involve changes in labor management but incur little increased cost and facilities or equipment. Other steps may involve capital investments, and the dairy producer must see a high likelihood for a positive economic impact to be willing to implement these steps.

For dairies that choose not to implement a testing program that identifies infectious cows, maternity management and newborn calf rearing practices can still be used to limit the likelihood of new infections. Such a program would focus on establishing conditions of impeccable hygiene for newborn calves. Practices that can be implemented include individual calving pens or a very clean, dry, and low-population-density multiple-use calving area, plus removal of calves immediately or within 1 hour after birth. Teats should be washed before colostrum collection, colostrum should be fed from individual cows to individual calves, the highest standards of hygiene should be used for calf workers and calf-rearing facilities, and pasteurized milk or milk replacer should be fed to baby calves. All of these practices decrease the likelihood that an individual calf is exposed to MAP from infected cows.

Use of individual cow test results enhances the ability to prevent exposure of baby calves to MAP. Strategically testing so that test results are available before cows enter the maternity area allows producers to segregate cows. Test-positive cows should be precluded from the maternity area and their colostrum or any later lactation waste milk should not be fed to calves. Producers who have excluded fecal culture-positive cows from the maternity area can achieve environmental fecal culture-negative status in this area and substantially reduce the potential for exposure of calves to MAP. Individual cow testing also provides the opportunity to selectively remove heifer calves born to test-positive cows from the herd. Such calves have a high risk of infection at birth because of the potential for in utero transfer and fecal contamination during the birthing process, even when other aspects of hygiene and colostrum management are well implemented.

For postweaning heifers, attention to environmental hygiene and exclusion of feeds that may have been contaminated by manure from adult cows are important aspects of a good JD control program. As animals age, the risk decreases that exposure to MAP will result in infection that eventuates in JD or positive fecal shedding status. Therefore, priority for control procedures should first be directed toward decreasing exposure of newborn calves.

TEST-AND-CULL

Management procedures that limit exposure of susceptible animals to MAP are more effective at reducing disease prevalence than simply testing and culling all MAP-infected cows. Therefore, the major emphasis in a good dairy herd JD control program is appropriately placed on procedures designed to limit calf exposure to MAP. It is undeniable, however, that eliminating MAP-infected/contagious animals from the herd is a powerful means to accomplish this end. Using the multiple hurdles concept, it is easy to see that decreasing the number of animals shedding MAP on the premise enhances the efficacy of every other control procedure by decreasing the overall MAP load on the farm.

It is important for a producer to evaluate the benefit of investing money in testing. For a dairy that has the opportunity to selectively remove cows from the herd, using diagnostic test results to identify cows for removal is a major benefit in JD control. This decision has to be carefully weighed against the benefit of maintaining those cows as producing animals. Although it has been clearly demonstrated that test-positive cows perform at suboptimal levels, many test positive cows maintain body weight and continue to return net positive revenue to the herd via milk production. A strict cash-flow evaluation of culling all test-positive animals will show this approach to be financially detrimental because the revenue the cow generates is lost and the cow needs to be replaced in the herd.[8] Therefore, many dairy producers prefer to keep MAP-infected cows in the herd and try to develop management procedures to minimize the impact such cows have on MAP transmission. Such mitigation measures may include keeping these cows out of the main maternity pen when they get ready to calve, selling their heifer offspring, identifying them as cows that are never bred again so that they produce milk but do not deliver calves in the future, and restricting their milk and colostrum from use to feed calves.

The question about culling test-positive animals should be carefully considered with the producer. While the management tactics presented above can reduce risk of MAP transmission from these cows, the producer needs to consider that these methods will not lower MAP transmission risk as effectively as will removing them from the herd. The producer should also consider whether these procedures will be uniformly and effectively implemented and what the downside risks are for a breach of protocol. If the cow has other liabilities such as other disease events, she may not be as productive as predicted. If the goal is to reduce probability of new MAP infections, then maintaining MAP fecal shedding cows in the herd is counterproductive. Further, if one of the goals of the JD control program is to increase success in heifer rearing, then there may be value in setting goals for heifer replacements that provide a time point when MAP-infected cows can be removed and replaced cost effectively.

PREVENTING INTRODUCTION OF NEW INFECTION

Preventing the introduction of MAP-infected cows into the herd is one of the greatest challenges in modern dairy herd management. Most producers that buy herd replacements from outside sources fail to enforce common biosecurity practices designed to prevent entry of a wide variety of pathogens, including bovine virus diarrhea, mastitis pathogens, Salmonella, or MAP. Given the distribution and prevalence of MAP infection in US dairy herds, buying replacements virtually ensures the introduction of MAP-infected animals unless methods are enforced to prevent entry. The best means of accomplishing this goal would be to close the herd and grow the herd only from internal replacements. This will require that cow health is sufficient to minimize cow removal and that heifer health is sufficient to provide enough replacements, which are good goals for every operation and should be seen as part of the overall JD control plan.

When replacement animals must be purchased, it is important that the producer understands the limitations of currently available tests. None of the current tests performed on individual animals can ensure freedom of MAP infection. Sources of animals can be prioritized to minimize risk of introduction of MAP to the herd (see Diagnostics article by Collins elsewhere in this issue). The national JD control program was devised with specific focus on developing protocols to identify low-risk herds.[11] The only reliable sources of infection-free animals are herds that have an established record of test-negative status.

REFERENCES

1. Lombard JE, Garry FB, McCluskey BJ, et al. Risk of removal and effects on milk production associated with paratuberculosis status in dairy cows. J Am Vet Med Assoc 2005;227(12):1975–81.

2. Villarino MA, Scott HM, Jordan ER. Influence of parity at time of detection of serologic antibodies to *Mycobacterium avium* subspecies paratuberculosis on reduction in daily and lifetime milk production in Holstein cows. J Anim Sci 2011;89(1):267–76.
3. USDA-APHIS-VS-CEAH. Johne's disease on U.S. dairies, 1991-2007. N521.0408, 1-4. Ft Collins (CO): USDA-APHIS-VS-CEAH; 2008. Available at: http://www.aphis.usda.gov/animal_health/nahms/dairy/downloads/dairy07/Dairy07_is_Johnes.pdf. Accessed August 18, 2011.
4. Nacy C, Buckley M. Mycobacterium avium paratuberculosis: Infrequent human pathogen or public health threat? Washington, DC: American Society for Microbiology; 2008.
5. Whitlock RH. Paratuberculosis control measures in the USA. In: Behr MA, Collins DM, editors. Paratuberculosis: Organism,disease, control. Oxfordshire. UK: CAB International; 2010. p. 319–9.
6. Risk Assessment. Handbook for Veterinarians and Dairy Producers. A guide for Johne's disease risk assessment and managment plans for dairy herds. Riverdale (MD): USDA; 2003. p. 1–8.
7. Collins MT, Gardner IA, Garry FB, et al. Consensus recommendations on diagnostic testing for the detection of paratuberculosis in cattle in the United States. J Am Vet Med Assoc 2006;229(12):1912–9.
8. Dorshorst NC, Collins MT, Lombard JE. Decision analysis model for paratuberculosis control in commercial dairy herds. Prev Vet Med 2006;75:92–122.
9. Wells SJ, Whitlock RH, Wagner BA, et al. Sensitivity of test strategies used in the Voluntary Johne's Disease Herd Status Program for detection of *Mycobacterium paratuberculosis* infection in dairy cattle herds. J Am Vet Med Assoc 2002;220(7):1053–7.
10. Bernard D. Developing and implementing HACCP in the USA. Food Control 2004;9(2-3):91–5.
11. USDA-APHIS. Uniform program standards for the voluntary bovine Johne's disease control program (APHIS 91-45-016). USDA-APHIS. APHIS 91-45-016. Ft Collins (CO): USDA-APHIS-VS-CEAH; 2010. Available at: http://www.aphis.usda.gov/animal_health/animal_diseases/johnes/downloads/johnes-ups.pdf. Accessed August 18, 2011.

Control of Paratuberculosis in Small Ruminants

Suelee Robbe-Austerman, DVM, MS, PhD

KEYWORDS
- Paratuberculosis • Johne's disease
- *Mycobacterium avium* subsp. *paratuberculosis* • Sheep
- Goats • Small ruminants

Most North American veterinary practitioners diagnosing paratuberculosis in small ruminants will do so using clinical experience gained from cattle. While that experience is very useful, there are important differences in the clinical presentation, diagnosis, management, and economics of the disease in these animals. It is these differences that will be emphasized here.

The prevalence of Johne's disease (JD) in sheep and goats in the United States is unknown but widespread. The lack of standardized robust diagnostic tests and funding for research in small ruminants has contributed to this problem. Unlike cattle, where a clear difference in the herd-level prevalence between dairy and beef cattle herds is seen, herd type or purpose does not seem to affect herd/flock prevalence of *Mycobacterium avium* subsp. *paratuberculosis* (MAP) infections in small ruminants. The flocking instinct keeps sheep and goats in close contact with each other, and for management reasons they usually give birth in confinement. This allows ample opportunity for transmission of MAP, even in large range flocks.

THE BIOLOGY OF MAP INFECTIONS IN SHEEP AND GOATS

In the United States, there are approximately 110 million beef and dairy cattle but only 7 million sheep. Yet there is a marked difference in the MAP strains infecting cattle and sheep. Cattle strains of MAP have a broad host range and can readily be cultured in most diagnostic laboratories. Sheep strains of MAP tend to be less pathogenic to hosts other than to sheep. Also, the sheep strain is exceptionally fastidious and does not grow under most laboratory conditions used in the United States. Geographically, sheep and cattle populations are located in similar regions of the country. Although a large number of sheep producers also own cattle, sheep strains of MAP continue to predominate in sheep. This suggests that cattle strains do not naturally maintain or

The author has nothing to disclose.
Mycobacteria Brucella Section, Diagnostic Bacteriology Laboratory, National Veterinary Services Laboratories, United States Department of Agriculture, Animal Plant Health Inspection Service, Veterinary Services, 1920 Dayton Avenue, Ames, IA 50010, USA
E-mail address: Suelee.Robbe-Austerman@aphis.usda.gov

Vet Clin Food Anim 27 (2011) 609–620
doi:10.1016/j.cvfa.2011.07.007
0749-0720/11/$ – see front matter Published by Elsevier Inc.

propagate in sheep despite the obvious opportunities for exposure to and acquisition of cattle strains of MAP, and despite experimental evidence demonstrating cattle strains can infect and cause disease in sheep.[1,2] Similar observations of sheep strains being identified rarely in cattle have been made in Australia, where total sheep and cattle population numbers are reversed.[3] Experimental challenge studies have clearly shown that cattle are resistant to infection with sheep strains of MAP.[4] The cause for this species affinity is not known. The importance of these observations to producers and veterinarians is that cattle are not at great risk for developing clinical JD from sheep harboring sheep strains of MAP, whereas sheep can acquire cattle strains and get JD. And, if the source of infection is removed, cattle strains of MAP do not seem to maintain themselves in sheep populations.[5]

In Australia. where goats have been exposed to both sheep and cattle MAP strains, it appears that goats are readily infected with either strain, with cattle strains of MAP being more pathogenic to goats than the sheep strains.[6] In the United States, clinical experience indicates that cattle MAP strains predominate in goats. In situations where veterinarians and producers are assessing risk in multispecies livestock operations, it may be important to identify which MAP strain is causing disease to develop effective control strategies. Most diagnostic laboratories specializing in paratuberculosis culture will readily be able to perform this test from infected tissue or from a culture isolate.

HOST IMMUNE RESPONSE: SHEEP VERSUS GOATS

Robust studies directly comparing the immune response and susceptibility of sheep and goats to MAP infection have not been done. However, experimental studies on each species, combined with clinical observations, suggest some significant differences in the immune responses to MAP by sheep and goats.[2,4,6] Goats appear to have a stronger, earlier antibody response than sheep, suggesting that current serological tests may be more sensitive in this species.[7] The literature also suggests that goats are more susceptible to MAP infections and more likely to develop clinical JD than either sheep or cattle, with cattle being the most resistant to the development of clinical disease.[4] This is consistent with field observations where some goat flocks were reported to have impressively high prevalence rates.[8,9] Some cattle and sheep experimentally challenged with MAP appear to clear the organism and be tissue and fecal culture negative. While this likely occurs in field situations, it is not known how often true recovery from an MAP infection occurs.[4]

Breed Susceptibility

In Australia, it has long been observed that Merino sheep are more susceptible to paratuberculosis infections than are cross-bred meat breeds.[10,11] However, genetic susceptibly may not be the primary contributing factor to this observation. One study directly measuring breed susceptibly reported only a 3.49% mean lifetime MAP infection incidence in Romney ewes versus 4.78% in Merino ewes, bringing into question the effect of breed differences on the susceptibility to MAP infections.[12] Other explanations for this observation could be differences in farm management or production stress.

Observations by U.S. veterinarians suggest breed differences in MAP infection rates. While breed differences in MAP infection susceptibility are possible, it could be an artifact of a large MAP-infected seedstock producer marketing sheep, thereby impacting a specific breed. Alternatively, certain production systems that may enhance MAP transmission tend to be used more often with certain breeds, such as a prolific sheep breed using an accelerated lambing program.

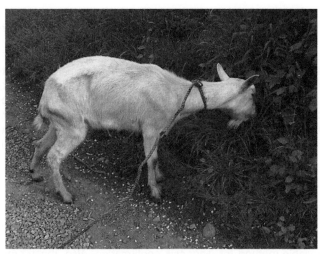

Fig. 1. Clinical paratuberculosis in a goat; low body condition but normal feces. (*Courtesy of* Michael T. Collins, DVM, PhD, Madison, WI.)

To date, no studies have examined breed susceptibility of paratuberculosis in goats. Although, similar to sheep, there are observational data suggesting certain breeds such as pygmy goats are more susceptible to infection, these observations must be confirmed with rigorously designed experimental challenge studies to ascertain if there are true breed susceptibility differences.

Diagnosing Paratuberculosis in Sheep and Goats

The classic clinical presentation of JD in cattle is a thin animal with profuse watery diarrhea and a good appetite. This is not the situation for sheep and goats. In these animals, if diarrhea occurs, it is usually intermittent and unremarkable; many times, infected animals are not identified or singled out for examination by the producer until they are ill enough to have a poor appetite. The most common clinical sign in sheep and goats is weight loss (**Fig. 1**). However, because many diseases cause nonspecific weight loss in small ruminants, it is nearly impossible to accurately diagnose paratuberculosis without laboratory diagnostics.[13] While weight loss is always present in clinical cases of JD, a broad variety of other clinical signs can occur: wool break, bottle jaw without severe anemia, and weakness. Because MAP infection alters the animals' immune system, animals with JD often also present with high parasite burdens. Finally, animals weakened by JD are more vulnerable to predator attacks.

It is not unusual for a small ruminant producer to be completely unaware of a paratuberculosis problem until the problem is severe or a cluster of younger animals (eg, 12 to 36 months old) becomes thin. Many external factors will influence the length of time between infection and manifestation of clinical signs in small ruminants. A larger exposure dose of MAP and stress tend to shorten the incubation period, and sheep or goats can present with clinical JD at a younger age than typically seen in cattle; it is not unusual to see JD before 12 months of age. Because clinical signs of JD are so nonspecific in small ruminants, MAP infections can exist in productive, well-managed, profitable herds/flocks for many years without detection. According to the US Department of Agriculture (USDA)'s NAHMS 2001 study of U.S. sheep flocks, of the 16.6% of sheep culled in 2000, 10.4% of them were culled or died because of progressive weight loss despite having normal appetite or common respiratory problems.[14] Therefore, veterinarians must be aware that culling animals with chronic unexplained weight loss routinely occurs in most sheep and goat flocks and herds, and often the underlying cause of this weight loss is undiagnosed.

If suspected, it is important to confirm MAP infection in a herd or flock that has not had previous JD-like cases confirmed by culture or polymerase chain reaction (PCR). This can be done through use of a necropsy and histologic examination, PCR, or culture of fecal or tissue samples. Occasionally, small ruminants can have disseminated mycobacterial infections due to mycobacteria other than MAP and they can be histologically similar to JD. Therefore, confirmation by culture or PCR is highly desirable.

Necropsy

Necropsy with histology and culture/PCR of tissues is the "gold standard" for confirmation of paratuberculosis. Unlike cattle, thin adult sheep and goats usually do not have a high market value. Therefore, on-farm necropsies of thin animals is an economically viable method for diagnosis confirmation. Also, many producers near large population centers will have consumers purchasing and slaughtering animals on the farm premises. In some situations, intestines from this type of activity may be available for examination. Unlike in cattle, where the hallmark gross lesion is a thickened intestine, particularly the terminal ileum, this finding is more subtle or absent in MAP-infected sheep and goats. Even clinically affected animals can also have grossly normal intestines. Nearly all clinical animals will have enlarged distal mesenteric lymph nodes (**Fig. 2**). For this reason, it is important for veterinarians to be familiar with the normal anatomy in order to recognize this common gross pathology. Even if the terminal ileum is grossly normal, veterinarians should sample the terminal ileum, incorporating the ileocecal junction and at least 5 cm of ileum as well as the distal mesenteric lymph nodes (half in formalin and half kept fresh for microbiology) for submission to a diagnostic laboratory.

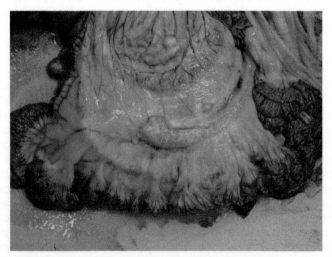

Fig. 2. Enlarged mesenteric lymph nodes typical of paratuberculosis in small ruminants. (*Courtesy of* Suelee Robbe-Austerman, DVM, MS, PhD, Ames, IA.)

Surveillance Testing

Occasionally, there is a need to classify the MAP infection status of a herd or flock, infected or test-negative. Testing options and strategies specific to small ruminants are discussed here and expanded on elsewhere in this issue.

Environmental fecal testing for flock and herd surveillance has great potential, but research to determine herd-level sensitivity and specificity has not been done; therefore, the number of samples and optimal sampling locations, such as near water troughs, feed troughs, barns, etc, and so on, have not been identified. Environmental fecal testing has the most potential for use in flocks and herds that are housed in a dry lot for an extended period of time, facilitating collection of fecal material that truly represents the adult flock. If the goal is to identify herds with greater than 2% MAP infection prevalence 95% of the time, the samples must collectively include fecal material from the vast majority of animals on the farm, unless the herd or flock is very large. In the author's experience, it is difficult to culture desiccated fecal material, so direct fecal PCR is recommended in lieu of culture on such samples.

Fecal pooling is more labor intensive than environmental fecal sampling, but fecal pooling ensures that animals are equally represented among samples and provides the ability to go back and test individual animals. At least 6 to 7 fecal pools should be tested per herd or flock and the actual number of animals in the pool can be varied depending on the herd-level diagnostic sensitivity needed.[15]

Surveillance by serology (enzyme-linked immunosorbent assay [ELISA]) requires testing a greater proportion of the herd/flock than by fecal testing. Although based on cattle, the tables in the diagnostics article in this issue give useful guidance for goats. Occasionally, ante mortem testing by serological methods is more convenient for the producer, such as using the milk ELISA for dairy goats. In sheep, it is generally not cost effective to serologically test clinically normal animals. Instead, sheep owners are advised to restrict serology to thin or cull ewes and rams (often called "tail enders") as a more cost-effective way to monitor a flock, initially with moderate sensitivity and accumulation of test results and over multiple years improves this further.

Slaughter surveillance, while not used in the United States, is the most important surveillance tool for paratuberculosis in small ruminants in Australia, especially in low prevalence areas. Inspectors examine the mesenteric lymph nodes and distal ileum of predominantly cull ewes and harvest samples from suspicious lesions. This method has good flock-level sensitivity, provided the inspector is adequately trained to recognize the somewhat subtle gross lesions of ovine paratuberculosis.[16,17] While it is very unlikely that a small ruminant slaughter surveillance program for paratuberculosis will be adopted in the United States, there may be unique individual situations where it is feasible to evaluate cull animals at slaughter and practitioners should capitalize on such opportunities.

Biosecurity: Preventing the Introduction of MAP to a Flock or Herd

For small ruminants, like all other species, paratuberculosis control starts with paratuberculosis prevention. One of the most important messages veterinarians can give to small ruminant producers is how to limit the risk of MAP introduction to herds/flocks. Veterinarians should provide both verbal biosecurity guidance and written educational materials, especially for new clients. A handout for sheep is available at http://farmandranchbiosecurity.com.[18] The single largest MAP infection risk is at the time of introduction of new animals. All too often, small ruminant producers experiencing disease problems forgot to consider the disease threat from acquiring a ram, teaser buck, or orphan kid. Testing the animals acquired is obvious but not sufficient. Knowing the MAP test status of the herd/flock of origin is most crucial.

Other MAP risks are generally much lower and have to do with the indirect exposure of a herd or flock to fecal material, such as pastures recently grazed by other small ruminants, cattle, or potentially wildlife or water runoff. If producers clearly understand the risks, they can make decisions that are in line with their goals and future plans.

Controlling Paratuberculosis

Sheep and goat operations are diverse, ranging from owners who view their animals as pets and attach a high emotional value to them, to producers managing multiemployee corporations and marketing branded products. Therefore, herd veterinarians must be flexible and innovative, clearly understanding owner's future goals, current production levels, facilities, and labor resources.

Because the investment to acquire sheep or goats is low, new owners with limited knowledge are common and veterinarians should have basic biosecurity and disease information readily available. There are several resources and handouts that veterinarians can provide or recommend specific to paratuberculosis.[19–22] Producers researching paratuberculosis in sheep or goats will likely encounter information from international sources. In other countries, vaccination against paratuberculosis is routinely used in small ruminants and is highly effective at reducing clinical disease. The vaccine available in the United States, Mycopar, is not approved for use in sheep and goats. And, based on limited experimental evidence, while effective, this vaccine can cause significant vaccine-induced tissue reactions if used at the dosage recommendations for cattle.

Control measures are discussed for 4 categories of small ruminant owners/operations: companion owners, commercial meat goat and sheep producers, commercial dairy goat and sheep producers, and seedstock producers. Admittedly, many producers and operations may fit into multiple categories.

Controlling Paratuberculosis: Companion Goats and Sheep

Typically, animals in these flocks/herds do not regularly produce kids or lambs. Many may be geriatric and are often not under much production stress, so animals with subclinical disease can survive a long time. When MAP infection is confirmed, the threat to the other sheep and goats on the farm is obvious. However, isolation of the MAP-infected animal is difficult; sheep and goats are not comfortable being housed alone. If culling is not an option for the owner, it may be possible to separate animals into high-risk and low-risk groups. Keep in mind that while young animals are the most susceptible to infection, small ruminants can be infected as adults and may succumb to JD at any age. Even though many companion sheep and goats are usually not in "high density" housing situations, they commonly stand in feed and water troughs, causing fecal contamination. Therefore, it is important that feeding systems such as keyhole feeders or other designs are used to keep animals from contaminating their feed and water.

It is not unusual for companion sheep and goat flocks to be composed of groups of highly related animals. This can have major consequences when paratuberculosis is diagnosed as paratuberculosis has a tendency to follow family lines, especially with goats. The owners may face a significant number of related animals succumbing to JD.

Individual animal testing may be appropriate for owners who consider their sheep or goats as companion animals. Currently, direct fecal PCR for sheep and culture or direct PCR for goats are the diagnostic tests best able to identify MAP-infected animals earliest in the course of infection (see diagnostics in this issue). A key concept that owners must understand is that negative tests do not ensure MAP freedom; multiple tests spaced over a long time will probably be required before the true non–MAP-infected status can be established.

Controlling Paratuberculosis: Commercial Meat Goats and Sheep

Flock veterinarians should not underestimate the emotional and financial impacts of a paratuberculosis diagnosis for a commercial herd or flock owner. Assure the individual that the disease can be controlled. The first step is to complete a risk assessment that evaluates the whole operation prior to issuing recommendations for changes in management or financial investments in testing. While there is not a risk assessment tool specifically designed for commercial meat goats and sheep in the United States, the beef cattle risk assessment tool provides a good template, with the inclusion of specific questions around thin ewe or doe management. Occasionally, the initial diagnosis of paratuberculosis occurs in recently purchased males or females. These animals tend to be under more stress than home-raised animals and consequently may break with clinical JD at a much higher rate than seen in the rest of the flock. In these cases, targeted testing of purchased animals may be warranted, and selection of replacement females from this population should be avoided. Depopulation of purchased animals may be advisable if the MAP infection rate is high and their exposure to the resident flock has been limited; the financial consequences of depopulation must be carefully considered.

For commercial flocks/herds, cost-benefit analysis on a paratuberculosis control program will have a significant impact on the decision-making process. Limited or targeted testing is best as one PCR test may be equivalent to 25% to 50% of the annual maintenance costs of a single ewe/doe. Permanent changes in facilities or management practices that reduce or eliminate the MAP transmission to replacement ewe lambs/does will have the greatest positive impact on control. Many commercial-operations control paratuberculosis and maintain profitability without diagnostic testing; however, targeted testing to identify the most infectious adults at strategic times during the year can be a cost-effective strategy that accelerates paratuberculosis control. Generally, the more intensive the management system, the more clinical JD is seen. In the author's experience, most sheep producers that have paratuberculosis in their flocks can keep their losses due to clinical JD to less than 5% of the adult flock and often maintain losses at less than 2%. If more than 5% of the adult flock is annually culled due to JD, a reassessment of management practices is needed. In instances where severe disease exists, depopulation may be the most economical option. In those cases, repopulation must be carefully considered as usually the conditions that allowed severe JD to develop still exist.

As discussed earlier, it appears that goats may be more susceptible to MAP infections than sheep, and serologic testing by ELISA is very effective at identifying clinical JD cases in goats. Pooled fecal PCR or culture, similar to what is recommended for beef cattle, may be useful to identify subclinically MAP-infected goats; however, the consulting veterinarian should be aware that because capital investments are so much lower for meat goats, the cost-benefit ratio of testing in goat herds can be dramatically different than that for cattle, even if the tests are equally accurate.

While reducing the culling rate due to paratuberculosis is the goal, an alteration of culling to remove chronically thin animals early may be one of the most important management changes that can be implemented. Producers often choose to cull at weaning time, but this may not be the optimal time to identify thin animals for culling, as high performing ewes and does can be also be a significant portion of this population. Instead, culling thin animals after shearing in winter time lambing systems or at 1 to 2 months prior to lambing or kidding can potentially reduce the number of animals shedding MAP. Although many producers are reluctant to cull ewes or does at this time, since most of the production costs have already incurred, doing so will lessen the exposure of young lambs and kids to the disease. Also, lambing is one of the most stressful labor-intensive times of the year; eliminating thin ewes that have a high risk of having small weak lambs will reduce the high labor inputs associated with these animals. Even if a program of testing or culling thin ewes and does prior to lambing is implemented, thin poor-doing animals will appear at various times during the year. Because the value of individual animals is relatively low, most producers are reluctant to take the time to market them individually. Implementing a system that removes these sporadically occurring thin animals early can pay dividends by reducing the MAP bioburden on the farm.

Because grazing is such a critical part of most meat goat and sheep operations, it is important to discuss the risks of acquiring paratuberculosis from pastures with the producer. The MAP organism can survive in pastures for over 1 year, but infectivity is substantially reduced within a few months.[23] It is important to educate the producer not to spread manure from the lambing/kidding sheds and dry lots directly onto pastures if they will be used for grazing in the same growing season. In certain regions of the country, the productivity of the soil and annual rainfall or irrigation allow animal stocking densities so high that small ruminants can easily be exposed to massive quantities of MAP simply by grazing.[24,25] In those regions of the country that have the parasite *Haemonchus*, a rough association can be made: if parasites are a significant problem, stocking densities are high enough for significant MAP transmission to occur by grazing. Other areas of the country, such as high mountain irrigated pastures, will not have this association. Because of the MAP host strain differences between cattle and sheep discussed earlier, alternate grazing of pastures with beef cattle or stockers and sheep (not goats) may be a more effective way to maximize productivity of pastures and reduce both parasite risks and MAP transmission risks. Meat goat herds that are used primarily to control brush or noxious weeds rather than to maximize the harvest of improved pastures are at low risk for transmitting paratuberculosis during the grazing season, providing they are able to meet their nutrient requirements with browse. This is also true for range flocks migrating during the summer. In these situations, the critical time for MAP exposure is during confined lambing or kidding. Ponds and dugouts are also potential areas for transmission.[26] If water sources on pastures have a significant potential to collect run-off from pastures and dry lots, consider providing a well water source. If that is not feasible, it may be worthwhile to fence off the pond, allowing for a grass buffer and pipe water from the pond to a holding tank. Other potential management changes or critical control points in a commercial sheep or meat goat operation are listed in **Table 1**.

Controlling Paratuberculosis: Dairy Goat and Sheep Operations

Fortunately, there are well-accepted "best management practices" for dairy goat and sheep operations to control caprine arthritis encephalitis (CAE) or ovine progressive pneumonia (OPP), and *Mycoplasma*.[27-29] These same practices are also important for paratuberculosis control. Dairies that employ an effective CAE/OPP/*Mycoplasma* control program rarely have significant problems with paratuberculosis; those that manage their dairies without at least some variation of the steps outlined here will likely experience other disease problems in addition to paratuberculosis. Key steps in these programs include prevention of newborns ingesting colostrum by taping teats or using "bras" or immediate kid/lamb removal; housing kids and lambs in a clean

Table 1
Additional critical control points and steps to reduce MAP exposure for small ruminants

Critical Control Points	Risk Reduction Measures
Creep areas	• Bed heavy to reduce manure exposure. • Design or alter feed troughs to prevent lambs or kids from standing in troughs. • Desirable location for creep—reduce lambs' kids from consuming waste feed from adults' feeding grounds by making the creep area a desirable location.
Replacement females	• After weaning, maintain replacement females separate from adults for as long as possible, preferably until lambing or kidding. • Avoid grazing replacement female animals in areas where mature animals graze.
Rams and bucks	• Isolate purchased rams and bucks except during breeding. • It is preferable for them to be maintained on premises that do not house animals from the main flock at anytime. • Consider testing the dams of purchased rams or bucks for paratuberculosis.
Grazing	• Rotational grazing methods that reduce parasite burdens will also reduce the exposure to MAP. • If ponds or dugouts are used for a water source, consider fencing these off and providing the water in troughs.
Dry lot management	• Reduce standing water, improve drainage, and consider constructing and maintaining mounds. • Evaluate feed trough designs to prevent stepping or standing in them and feed spillage on the ground. • If feeding on the ground, select areas that do not have visible fecal material. • Maintain clean water troughs.
Lambing or kidding	• Keep moisture levels low in barns if lambing or kidding indoors. • Keep bedding sufficiently deep to prevent dirty teats. • Identify potential replacement females so that they can be traced back to their dams in case their dams become clinically positive or test positive.

environment separate from adults, heat-treating colostrum; pasteurizing milk fed to kids or using milk replacer; and separating replacement females from adults until the first kidding or lambing. Therefore, if veterinarians are investigating a paratuberculosis problem on a small ruminant dairy, it is important to recognize that paratuberculosis may be an indicator disease and other economically important diseases are probably posing a threat to the operation as well. A broad disease control approach is essential for these cases.

It is important for the veterinary practitioner to spend time discussing the heat-treatment of colostrum with the producer. Heat-treating colostrum for the recommended 133°–138°F (56°–59°C) for 60 minutes is not sufficient to completely kill all MAP, although it drastically reduces their number.[30] A significant effort has been made in both cattle and small ruminants to identify a temperature/time combination that will totally eliminate MAP, preserve immunoglobulins, and keep colostrum from becoming too viscous to feed.[31–34] Colostrum from small ruminants is so variable in initial viscosity that identifying a best time-temperature combination may not be possible; going above 59°C will increase the number of batches ruined. Instead, promote heat-treatment of colostrum at the standard temperatures as a partially protective measure that must be combined with efforts to identify and remove clinically affected adults as the most reasonable approach. Veterinarians should offer to quality check pasteurizers and on-farm thermometers to ensure they are performing as expected. Pasteurization of surplus and waste milk for kid consumption should be handled differently than colostrum; pasteurization temperatures should be higher. For batch pasteurizers, the milk should be heated to 63°C for 30 minutes (low-temperature long-time [LTLT] pasteurization) or 162°F (72°) for 15 seconds (high-temperature short-time [HTST] pasteurization). Again, it must be emphasized to the producer that these systems require maintenance and regular calibration to ensure proper performance.

Use of diagnostic tests helps identify the most significant sources of infection for culling, which helps accelerate paratuberculosis control. In goats, ELISAs work well and the testing programs effective for dairy cattle will perform similarly in goats. For sheep, serology is less effective.

Controlling Paratuberculosis: Seedstock Operations

The major difference between commercial and seedstock operations is the economic feasibility of testing, and a potential goal of eradication. Effective diagnostic test methods for sheep are quite limited. The antibody tests, AGID, and ELISA do not work as well in sheep as they do in cattle and goats, and, as mentioned previously, and most laboratories are using culture methods that do not support the growth and detection of sheep strains. This ultimately leaves direct fecal PCR as the diagnostic testing method of choice. Testing animals either individually or in pools just prior to lambing is a good approach. For goats, following the testing protocols recommended for seedstock dairy and beef cattle producers is recommended.

Producers should understand that while these testing methods can dramatically reduce the prevalence of paratuberculosis, they are unlikely to eradicate the disease without more drastic management changes. Sheep flocks can test negative by individual whole herd testing and still be able to transmit MAP infections to the next generations without being detected. Eradication steps may include practicing lamb and kid removal similar to CAE/OPP control programs, heat treating colostrum from individual test-negative dams, and rearing these lambs at a second "clean" location using milk replacer. This second location can be used to develop a "clean" flock and then the original location can be depopulated. This of course is a drastic, expensive protocol. Sheep and goat producers should be committed to practicing strict biosecurity if they go through this process. With goats, artificial insemination is routine and semen is readily available. Sheep producers still need to introduce rams or use laparoscopic artificial insemination, which, while feasible, is expensive.

REFERENCES

1. Kluge JP, Merkal RS, Monlux WS, et al. Experimental paratuberculosis in sheep after oral, intratracheal, or intravenous inoculation lesions and demonstration of etiologic agent. Am J Vet Res 1968;29(5):953–62.
2. Stewart DJ, Vaughan JA, Stiles PL, et al. A long-term study in Merino sheep experimentally infected with Mycobacterium avium subsp. paratuberculosis: clinical disease, faecal culture and immunological studies. Vet Microbiol 2004;104(3–4): 165–78.
3. Moloney BJ, Whittington RJ. Cross species transmission of ovine Johne's disease from sheep to cattle: an estimate of prevalence in exposed susceptible cattle. Austral Vet J 2008;86(4):117–23.

4. Stewart DJ, Vaughan JA, Stiles PL, et al. A long-term bacteriological and immunological study in Holstein-Friesian cattle experimentally infected with Mycobacterium avium subsp. paratuberculosis and necropsy culture results for Holstein-Friesian cattle, Merino sheep and Angora goats. Vet Microbiol 2007;122(1–2):83–96.

5. Whittington RJ, Taragel CA, Ottaway S, et al. Molecular epidemiological confirmation and circumstances of occurrence of sheep (S) strains of Mycobacterium avium subsp. paratuberculosis in cases of paratuberculosis in cattle in Australia and sheep and cattle in Iceland. Vet Microbiol 2001;79(4):311–22.

6. Stewart DJ, Vaughan JA, Stiles PL, et al. A long-term study in Angora goats experimentally infected with Mycobacterium avium subsp. paratuberculosis: clinical disease, faecal culture and immunological studies. Vet Microbiol 2006;113(1–2): 13–24.

7. Whittington RJ, Eamens GJ, Cousins DV. Specificity of absorbed ELISA and agar gel immuno-diffusion tests for paratuberculosis in goats with observations about use of these tests in infected goats. Austral Vet J 2003;81(1–2):71–5.

8. Manning EJ, Steinberg H, Krebs V, et al. Diagnostic testing patterns of natural Mycobacterium paratuberculosis infection in pygmy goats. Can J Vet Res 2003;67(3): 213–8.

9. Gezon HM, Bither HD, Gibbs HC, et al. Identification and control of paratuberculosis in a large goat herd. Am J Vet Res 1988;49(11):1817–23.

10. Morris CA, Hickey SM, Henderson HV. The effect of Johne's disease on production traits in Romney, Merino and Merino x Romney-cross ewes. N Z Vet J 2006;54(5): 204–9.

11. Lugton IW. Cross-sectional study of risk factors for the clinical expression of ovine Johne's disease on New South Wales farms. Aust Vet J Jun 2004;82(6):355–65.

12. Hickey SM MC, Dobbie JL, Lake DE. Heritability of Johne's disease and survival data from Romney and Merino sheep. Proc N Z Soc Anim Prod 2003;63:179–82.

13. Sherman DM. Unexplained weight loss in sheep and goats. A guide to differential diagnosis, therapy, and management. Vet Clin North Am Large Anim Pract 1983;5(3): 571–90.

14. Sheep 2001, part II: reference of sheep health in the United States, 2001–2003. Available at: http://www.aphis.usda.gov/animal_health/nahms/sheep/downloads/sheep01/Sheep01_dr_PartII.pdf. Accessed November 10, 2010.

15. Dhand NK, Sergeant E, Toribio J-ALML, et al. Estimation of sensitivity and flock-sensitivity of pooled faecal culture for Mycobacterium avium subsp. paratuberculosis in sheep. Prev Vet Med 2010;95(3–4):248–57.

16. Abbott KA, Whittington RJ. Monte Carlo simulation of flock-level sensitivity of abattoir surveillance for ovine paratuberculosis. Prev Vet Med 2003;61(4):309–32.

17. Bradley TL, Cannon RM. Determining the sensitivity of abattoir surveillance for ovine Johne's disease. Aust Vet J 2005;83(10):633–6.

18. Biosecurity in Practice Series: Sheep flocks, a guide to biosecurity in sheep production. Farm and Ranch Biosecurity. Available at: http://www.farmandranchbiosecurity.com/Sheep_Insert.pdf. Accessed December 28, 2010.

19. OJD: disease risk management 2008; PRIMEFACT 667. Available at: http://www.dpi.nsw.gov.au/__data/assets/pdf_file/0004/225094/OJD-disease-risk-management.pdf. Accessed December 28, 2010.

20. Ovine Johne's disease (OJD). 2008; PRIMEFACT 661. Available at: http://www.dpi.nsw.gov.au/__data/assets/pdf_file/0011/223994/Ovine-johnes-disease-OJD.pdf. Accessed December 28, 2010.

21. National Johne's Education Initiative, National Institute for Animal Agriculture. Available at: http://www.johnesdisease.org/. Accessed December 28, 2010.

22. Johne's Information Center. Available at: http://johnes.org/. Accessed December 28, 2010.
23. Whittington RJ, Marshall DJ, Nicholls PJ, et al. Survival and dormancy of *Mycobacterium avium* subsp. *paratuberculosis* in the environment. Appl Environ Microbiol 2004;70(5):2989–3004.
24. Reddacliff LA, Whittington RJ. Experimental infection of weaner sheep with S strain *Mycobacterium avium* subsp. *paratuberculosis*. Vet Microbiol 2003;96(3):247–58.
25. Reddacliff LA, McGregor H, Abbott K, et al. Field evaluation of tracer sheep for the detection of early natural infection with *Mycobacterium avium* subsp *paratuberculosis*. Austral Vet J 2004;82(7):426–33.
26. Whittington RJ, Marsh IB, Reddacliff LA. Survival of *Mycobacterium avium* subsp. *paratuberculosis* in dam water and sediment. Appl Environ Microbiol 2005;71(9):5304–8.
27. Rowe JD, East NE. Risk factors for transmission and methods for control of caprine arthritis-encephalitis virus infection. Vet Clin North Am Food Anim Pract 1997;13(1):35–53.
28. Dawson M. Caprine arthritis-encephalitis. In Pract 1987;9:8–11.
29. MacKenzie RW, Oliver RE, Rooney JP, et al. A successful attempt to raise goat kids free of infection with caprine arthritis encephalitis virus in an endemically infected goat herd. N Z Vet J 1987;35(11):184–6.
30. Meylan M, Rings DM, Shulaw WP, et al. Survival of *Mycobacterium paratuberculosis* and preservation of immunoglobulin G in bovine colostrum under experimental conditions simulating pasteurization. Am J Vet Res 1996;57(11):1580–5.
31. McMartin S, Godden S, Metzger L, et al. Heat treatment of bovine colostrum. I: effects of temperature on viscosity and immunoglobulin G level. J Dairy Sci 2006;89(6):2110–8.
32. Fernández A, Ramos JJ, Loste A, et al. Influence of colostrum treated by heat on immunity function in goat kids. Comp Immunol Microbiol Infect Dis 2006;29(5–6):353–64.
33. Argüello A, Castro N, Capote J, et al. Effects of refrigeration, freezing-thawing and pasteurization on IgG goat colostrum preservation. Small Rumin Res 2003;48(2):135–9.
34. Godden SM, Smith S, Feirtag JM, et al. Effect of on-farm commercial batch pasteurization of colostrum on colostrum and serum immunoglobulin concentrations in dairy calves. J Dairy Sci 2003;86(4):1503–12.

Paratuberculosis in Captive and Free-Ranging Wildlife

Elizabeth J.B. Manning, MPH, MBA, DVM

KEYWORDS

• Exotic • Johne's disease • Nonruminant • Ruminant
• Paratuberculosis • Wildlife • Zoo

This chapter addresses the special issues pertaining to *Mycobacterium avium* subsp. *paratuberculosis* (MAP) infection, surveillance, diagnosis, management, and control for captive and free-ranging ruminant hoofstock, plus a short review of MAP infection in nonruminant species.

While the majority of Johne's disease cases are concentrated in domestic agriculture ruminant species (cattle, sheep, goats, etc., as addressed elsewhere in this issue), the extensive host range for this infection is also documented in nondomestic, or "exotic," hoofstock. Although cases may not yet have been recorded in each and every species of the taxonomic suborder Ruminantia (and their camelid cousins), it is clear the ruminant host range is broad: from anoa to zebu. In fact, all ruminants, whether free-ranging or captive, are believed susceptible to infection by MAP and by all strains of MAP. The core epidemiologic and pathologic facets of the infection are generally the same across ruminant species—newonatal infection, intermittent shedding in feces and milk, late onset of fatal clinical disease characterized by granulomatous infiltration of the proximal gastrointestinal tract and associated lymph nodes.

There is no strong evidence to date of significant differences in susceptibility across ruminant species. The higher prevalence of Johne's disease seen in, for example, a closely held infected bovine dairy herd versus a population of free-ranging tule elk is not due to greater innate predisposition to MAP infection in cattle. Instead, it arises from higher animal density (more cows per acre) and subsequently greater MAP environmental contamination than what are typically the case for an elk range. Since prevalence is largely a function of infection pressure and since dairy bovid calves are more exposed to MAP than are free-ranging cervid calves, the frequency of transmission due to exposure is greater in the dairy herd. Beef cattle operations report a much lower prevalence, in keeping with the industry's range-based lower stocking density.[1] With the continued loss of habitat and the narrowing of the barrier

---

The author has nothing to disclose.
a. Prionics Parachek, Zurich, Switzerland.
Johne's Information Center, School of Veterinary Medicine, University of Wisconsin–Madison, 2015 Linden Drive, Madison, WI 53706, USA
E-mail address: emanning@wisc.edu

Vet Clin Food Anim 27 (2011) 621–630
doi:10.1016/j.cvfa.2011.07.008
0749-0720/11/$ – see front matter © 2011 Elsevier Inc. All rights reserved.

vetfood.theclinics.com

between free-ranging wildlife and farmed animals however, free-ranging wildlife exposure to MAP may increase, in which case the prevalence is expected to rise.

Once introduced, the prevalence of MAP infections in intensively managed wildlife populations (such as farmed deer)[2] mirrors what is seen for other closely held ruminants. For ruminant wildlife, exposure to the organism in the first few months of life is a primary risk factor. The level of risk is affected by population density and close association with water and range contaminated by heavily infected, usually domestic agriculture, herds.[3,4]

CAPTIVE WILDLIFE

Detection and control of MAP infection is challenging in any hoofstock operation, but the particular constraints of caring for a zoologic collection increase the challenge. These often rare, and rarely handled, hoofstock species are managed to serve several purposes: emblems of endangered species conservation, a source for genetic material, and subjects of both education and entertainment. The sale of healthy animals among collections may be a substantial source of revenue for the zoo. These purposes sometimes conflict with biosecurity policies and complicate control of infectious diseases.

Hoofstock susceptible to MAP infection are important members of zoo collections for a majority of institutions accredited by the American Association of Zoo and Aquaria (AZA). AZA-accredited zoos meet high standards of sanitation, animal care, environmental enrichment, record keeping, and facility maintenance. Dedicated technical and keeper staff can provide accurate enclosure, herd, breeding, and individual animal health histories. These personnel should be considered valuable resources when assessing the risk factors for MAP transmission, as should the extensive online databases that track all aspects of each animal's handling and treatment. There are numerous, usually smaller, non–AZA-accredited game parks that can benefit from Johne's disease risk assessment as well.

Prevalence

As reported in 2001, up to one-third of zoos accredited by the AZA Association reported a minimum of 1 MAP-infected animal since 1995. The majority of these cases were in domestic species, but a significant incidence in exotic species has been reported as well.[5,6] Current prevalence estimates are not available, but MAP infection should be on a differential diagnosis list for any adult ruminant with weight loss.

Risk Factors

The primary risk factor for *introducing* MAP infection to a zoologic collection is bringing in an undetected infection from another zoo (exotic species) or from a local herd for farm or "petting zoo" exhibits (domestic agriculture species). The primary risk factors for *spreading* the infection are vertical transmission from an infected dam, or ingestion at a susceptible age of grass, feed, or water contaminated by MAP-laden manure from an infected enclosure-mate.

Due to the operational constraints of most zoos, and in some cases the lack of familiarity with Johne's disease, one may encounter on the same premise both strictly controlled and completely unaddressed risk factors. On the one hand, you may find that all enclosures are raked daily and manure composted ("zoo doo" is a popular fertilizer), water and feed troughs are cleaned regularly, and breeding and health histories are well documented. On the other hand, standing and drinking water may recirculate through numerous exhibits, enclosure sod may have been cut from dairy cattle pastures, and newborn hoofstock may be bottle-fed unpasteurized colostrum and milk purchased from an untested local dairy.

The central topics for MAP risk assessment universal to domestic agriculture herds also pertain to these special populations:

- Fecal-oral exposure to MAP for young animals
  - Evaluate breeding program in light of MAP transmission.
  - Evaluate calving/kidding/lambing pen sanitation.
  - Evaluate preweaning and postweaning sanitation.
  - Evaluate adult manure contamination of water, feed, and environment.

Once the usual risk factors have been assessed, however, the subsequent management plan may diverge significantly from what is commonly outlined for domestic ruminant herds because:

- Sample collection/examination is difficult and dangerous for the animal (knock-down and sedation)
- Institutions may not be able to cull test-positive/infected animal
  - Highpublic profile animals
  - Genetic value
- Lack of validated serologic assays
- Limited space for quarantine, separation of test-positives from test-negatives
- Inability to redesign enclosure, water system
- No clinical, breeding, MAP exposure history for animals purchased from private hoofstock dealers.

For a management plan to be effective in limiting transmission, it must take into account the particulars of zoo animal husbandry and recognize the restrictions under which they operate.

Surveillance

Hoofstock are usually kept in mixed species enclosures typical of regional habitats (ie, Eastern Africa Savanna: bongo, impala, and giraffe), and many are brought into a barn nightly. Even so, hoofstock often must be chased, driven into a squeeze cage, or completely knocked down and sedated in order for diagnostic samples to be collected. Many zoos do not have adequate facilities to safely capture and contain hoofstock while samples are collected; capture stress and myopathy are serious concerns for both the animal and its enclosure-mates. This means samples may be obtained on an opportunistic basis only (hoof-trimming or dental procedures, transfer to another exhibit, treatment for another clinical illness). Opportunistic sampling should be done at every opportunity, freezing serum (–20 or –80 centigrade) and direct rectal manure (–80) for later testing if necessary.

Some AZA facilities monitor their hoofstock on a regular basis for MAP infection, inspired perhaps by a prior confirmed case of Johne's disease or a desire to ensure that the animals in their public contact areas are free of the infection. However, since hoofstock are handled infrequently, zoo budgets are limited, and animal health resources are often focused on urgent issues, screening for MAP infection is often a low priority. For the majority of zoologic institutions, the primary goad for assessing hoofstock for MAP infection, apart from clinical disease, is the prospect of shipping an animal to another collection. These shipments (requested for endangered species breeding purposes, or by recipient zoo curators to augment the appeal of the collection, or to rid themselves of excess numbers of a particular species after a successful breeding program) usually trigger a raft of diagnostic tests, often including some sort of check for MAP infection.

The most valuable piece of diagnostic information for MAP control is the infection status of the adult animals in the enclosure (a zoo's version of a "herd") supplying the animal to be shipped. This information is often not available, however, at the time a curator notifies the veterinarian that a hoofstock shipment is being planned. Instead, a common preshipment assay choice (based on the proceedings of a widely attended workshop focused on Johne's disease in zoos)[7] is culture of 3 fecal samples, collected from the ground some days apart as feasible for the enclosure staff (keeper) schedule. Unfortunately, the speed of animal transfer once approved often outpaces the 7-week incubation period (liquid culture; solid media culture requires 16 weeks or more before a "test-negative" result is released). Potentially infected animals thus may shipped thousands of miles and perhaps even released from quarantine before a result is received. In the absence of the enclosure infection status and the health/infection status of the dam, this "preship" protocol is of limited value.

The following are additional reasons captive wildlife managers choose to test portions of or all of their collections:

1. Confirm diagnosis in individual animals with clinical signs
2. Establish enclosure infection status before breeding or introducing young animals
3. Screen local source herd before bringing in sheep, goats, or cattle to a farm exhibit or camels for rides
4. Determine if a positive result on a tuberculosis test is actually due to infection by MAP vs a member of the *M. tuberculosis* complex (antigenic cell wall components are shared across many mycobacterial species, making cross reactions in immunologic tests possible)
5. Ensure milk for bottle-rearing comes from an uninfected dam
6. Ensure embryo-recipient animal is not infected
7. Screen for infection in feral/wild animals in parks that might carry MAP from enclosure to enclosure (raccoons, mice, etc).

There are 2 populations that must be considered separately for diagnostic purposes in the zoo setting: exotic vs domestic agriculture hoofstock. Many zoos manage farm or children's zoo exhibits that house more docile species for the public to touch and perhaps feed. Typically, these include sheep, goats, and cattle. All of these may be tested as outlined in other chapters of this book, focusing especially on finding animals that are shedding MAP. Of particular importance from a biosecurity perspective are the seasonal residents, brought in perhaps to kid or lamb during the spring and summer months and then sent back to the source herd. It is rare that the local source herds for these animals have been tested for Johne's disease or have any reliable health histories; they represent one of the greatest risks for contaminating zoo premises and should be high on the priority list for surveillance.

Once the reason(s) the zoo wishes to test for Johne's disease, a surveillance program that best meets its needs may be tailored. This program should outline the type of test, when to test, which animals to focus on, the cost of testing, and how to interpret the results. In a zoo collection, the type of program will depend on the collection's history of Johne's disease, breeding plans, budget, and whether and when animals are transferred in/out of the collection.

Clinical Diagnosis

As discussed elsewhere in this issue, there are 2 primary types of diagnostic tests: those that look for the organism that causes Johne's disease (MAP) and those that focus on the animal's response to infection by MAP (antibody in the blood or milk). Because a test-positive result can halt animal movements within and across zoo collections and block breeding programs for invaluable animals, false-positive results are extremely disruptive for this industry. Assay specificity is therefore crucial for either the initial screening test or the confirmatory assay.

Fecal culture is an effective, if not the best, choice for nondomestic species. Liquid culture may yield a MAP-positive result long before the 7-week incubation period needed before a sample is deemed negative for MAP. (The greater the number of MAP in a sample, the sooner a positive signal is produced.) Culture is also useful for tissues collected at necropsy and for environmental fecal samples collected in heavily trafficked areas to establish the contamination status of a premise. The laboratory may pool up to 5 fecal or environmental samples, thus reducing the cost to the institution without sacrificing too much diagnostic sensitivity. If a pool is culture-positive, the individual samples contributing to that pool are then tested. Only labs experienced in MAP isolation should be selected to process these samples (see NVSL annual proficiency test results at http://www.aphis.usda.gov/animal_health/lab_info_services/approved_labs.shtml.)

Several commercial direct PCRs have been validated for bovine fecal samples. The assays look for the presence of MAP's genetic material instead of the living organism. Most labs provide a result in less than 1 week. The sensitivities of culture and PCR are believed to be generally comparable. Be aware that false-positives can occur with PCRs (http://www.aphis.usda.gov/animal_health/lab_info_services/proficiency.shtml) and that the assay may not perform equally well with nonbovine manure due to biological inhibitors or sample matrix differences. Do not rely on PCR results only in making culling decisions. There have been unfortunate cases of unnecessary euthanasia of captive wildlife based on unreliable PCR results from inexperienced labs.

Previous generations of commercial ELISAs have been used effectively with nondomestic ruminant sera. Unfortunately, the ability of current commercial ELISA formulations to detect exotic species' immunoglobulin produced in response to MAP infection have not been published. Both false-negative (inability to detect the species IgG) and false-positive (cross-reacting antibody due to a different infection, such as *C. pseudotuberculosis* or a non-MAP mycobacteria) results may occur. The USDA has validated the ParaCheck ELISA (Prionics, Zurich, Switzerland) for use on milk or sera from cattle, sheep, and goats; it may have some utility for cervid species as well. While a positive ELISA result is not sufficiently specific to confirm a Johne's disease diagnosis in a nondomestic ruminant species, it does raise the index of suspicion.

Due to the slowly developing biology of MAP infection, it is only adult animals that produce the targets (analytes) needed by diagnostic tests. Calves, kids, lambs, etc are infected while very young, but they do not shed the organism with any frequency (therefore the organism detection assays will be negative), nor do they produce antibody (therefore the blood/milk tests will be negative). That is why it is recommended that diagnostic tests be used only for animals at least 18 months old. If a zoo wishes to introduce a young animal, to best determine its infection the dam should be tested for MAP infection and the infection status of the enclosure in which it was raised should be determined.

AZA-accredited zoos are required to perform a necropsy for any animal dying on the premises. The standard protocols include inspection of mesenteric lymph nodes and distal gastrointestinal tract for gross lesions consistent with Johne's disease. Cases of infection will be missed, however, if only the presence of gross lesions is relied on, either because the animal died too early in the stage of MAP infection for gross lesions to appear or because the animal belonged to a species frequently free of gross lesions even in late stage disease (sheep, perhaps bison). Effective surveillance for MAP at each ruminant necropsy should include acid-fast staining and microscopic inspection of the ileum and mesenteric lymph nodes as well as culture of these tissues plus feces. An additional post-mortem option is PCR targeted at MAP insertion sequences (hspX or IS900) using a scroll from formalin-fixed paraffin-embedded tissues. This assay is likely more sensitive if acid-fast rods are noted microscopically in tissues collected at a necropsy.

Resources

An excellent and extensive resource for all things ungulate can be found at: http://www.ultimateungulate.com/ designed and maintained by Brent Huffman, Toronto Zoo. This site is invaluable for ecologic, taxonomic, behavioral, and conservation information for any species one may encounter in a zoologic collection. Should you need to refresh your memory on the differences between pudu and Père David deer, this is the resource for you.

Membership in AZA provides a valuable network of greater than 6000 zoo and aquarium professionals, organizations, and suppliers worldwide. The AZA is the accrediting body for zoos and maintains extensive resources addressing wildlife conservation, education, science, and animal care (http://www.aza.org/). The accreditation manual is a good place to start for an overview of the elements of zoo collection management, care, and regulation. Expertise pertinent to veterinary concerns can be found amongst the members of the TAGs (Taxonomic Advisory Groups) and the SSPs (species survival plan programs).

The zoologic community maintains a sophisticated and extensive global online database to manage animal inventory (an estimated 2.3 million animals). Software produced by this organization supports a collection's medical records (MedArks, now ZIMS). This database tracks all elements of an animal's history from birth to death across participant institutions (825 member zoos, aquariums, and related organizations in 76 countries).

FREE-RANGING RUMINANTS

Currently, Johne's disease prevalence in free-ranging ruminants appears to be neither extensive on a herd basis nor geographically widely distributed. The catalogue of MAP infection in free-ranging ruminants is incomplete, however, due to sparse funding for surveillance plus the challenges of animal handling and sample collection. Valid estimates of disease prevalence in noncaptive populations can rarely be made since the majority of studies are necessarily completed on a "snapshot" basis at one point in time. While isolation of MAP has been reported for individual animals in a broad range of free-ranging ruminant species, much of these data come from retrospective studies based on MAP isolates in laboratory repositories.[8] These repository-based reports have expanded the list of potential host species but can show little about subsequent disease, transmission, incidence, or prevalence in free-ranging ruminant herds. The inability to trace epidemiologic factors over time (ie, to assess true infection vs "pass-through" from a contaminated environment, onset and rate of shedding, incidence in offspring, maintenance of the infection in the herd without reinfection from other infected species sharing range, etc) particularly restricts our understanding of this slow-to-develop infection in free-ranging wildlife.

The few exceptions to individual case reports are long-standing infections in a tule elk herd (CA), a subpopulation of key deer (FL), and a herd of bison composed of animals from multiple source herds (MT).[9–11]

MAP infection in elk is primarily represented by the population of tule elk (*Cervus elaphus nannodes*) at the Point Reyes National Seashore (PRNS) reserve where the first case was documented in 1979. The infection and clinical disease have been confirmed in adult animals since that time. Reserve managers do not currently report any obvious effect on herd health or reproduction in the approximately 450-animal herd due to Johne's disease; diagnostic testing is no longer part of the management plan (N. Gates, PORE, personal communication). No evidence of MAP infection has been found in native black-tailed deer also located at PRNS. No evidence of MAP infection was found in surveys of elk in Arkansas and Montana/Wyoming.[12,13]

White-tailed deer (*Odocoileus virginianus*) are a susceptible species; a multistate survey of wild white-tailed deer in southeastern United States found a very low prevalence of infection (0.3%).[14] One clinical case in a 2-year-old male white-tailed deer from Virginia was recently reported.[15] Johne's disease was first diagnosed in an endangered Florida Key deer (a subspecies of white-tailed deer; *Odocoileus virginianus clavium*) in 1996. Six additional Key deer were found to be infected from 1998 to 2004. Managers believe the organism persists in a portion of the Key deer population limited to a relatively small geographic area within their range.[16]

The principal bison population appearing in the literature was infected by a difficult-to-culture strain ("bison strain"). Since that time, cases of infection with the "cattle strain" of MAP have been reported in other bison populations (both captive and free-ranging). In addition, the "bison strain" was found to be the cause of Johne's disease in a dairy cow in Idaho, with anecdotal reports of this strain in a few free-ranging elk. In Canada, surveillance of bison with PCR of fecal samples produced positive results in several herds, but the organism was not recovered. A serologic survey of banked sera collected over multiple years from free-ranging bison managed in 4 Western national parks was completed under the auspices of the National Park Service. ELISA results for greater than 1200 serum samples did not indicate the presence of MAP infection in these populations (Manning, unpublished data).

Clinical Johne's disease has also been reported on occasion in Rocky Mountain bighorn sheep (*Ovis canadensis canadensis*), Rocky Mountain goats (*Oreamnos americanus*), as well as free-ranging red (*Cervus elaphus hippelaphus*) and fallow deer in Europe.[17] A recent report of free-ranging guanacos (*Lama guanicoe*) in Chile describes isolation of the MAP "cattle-strain" from fecal samples at a low prevalence (21 of 501).[18] Paratuberculosis in camelids under domestic husbandry has also been reported, including alpacas (*Lama pacos*) in Australia and camels (*Camelus dromedarius*) from Egypt and Saudi Arabia.

The majority of cases in ruminant wildlife are reported in animals sharing contaminated fields, range, or water[19] with MAP-infected domestic agriculture species. Given the volume of MAP-contaminated manure produced by high-prevalence herds of domestic stock, and the widespread use of the manure as field fertilizer, it is likely that the direction of infection pressure is from farmed livestock to free-ranging ruminants. (An infected cow may shed 10^6 CFU per gram of manure; experimental infection studies indicate that an infective oral dose for young ruminants is 4×10^6 CFU.[20])

However, the simple recovery of MAP in low numbers from an environmental sample does not ensure "spill-over" into ruminant wildlife and the creation of a reservoir of infection. The organisms (obligate pathogens believed incapable of replicating in the environment) must be swallowed in sufficient numbers in sufficient frequency by a susceptible animal at a vulnerable age (estimated to be <6 months old) to generate good odds that a new Johne's disease case will occur.

Few measures can be taken to prevent transmission of MAP in free-ranging species. Efforts should be made to keep herd density low, to minimize contact with domestic ruminant species (and their potentially contaminated fields and pastures), and to translocate wild ruminants only from test-negative populations if possible.

MAP infection does not yet appear to be a significant threat to free-ranging wildlife health. The threat may increase however due to increased infection pressure from rising prevalence in domestic livestock and dwindling wildlife habitat.

NONRUMINANT SPECIES

Subsequent to MAP's isolation from a nonruminant (rabbit) population sharing pastures with Johne's disease dairy cattle herds in Scotland, several detailed studies of the infected population have assessed important epidemiologic variables such as shared pastures with dairy cattle with Johne's disease, routes of transmission, local MAP strain pathogenicity, etc.[21,22] In contradistinction to this "hot spot," in other locales MAP isolations have been made only sporadically in low numbers from nonruminant animals such as the brown hare, brown rat and long-tailed field mouse, raccoons, opossums, armadillos, feral cats, and skunk.[4] Pathologic findings consistent with paratuberculosis including intracellular acid-fast bacteria are rarely seen in these species. Isolation of MAP with no indication of disease has also been the case in predator and scavenger species such as red fox, stoat, weasel, crows, rooks, and jackdaws. These infected predators and scavengers are described as "dead-end hosts" and do not constitute high-risk factors for interspecies transmission.[8] It is invalid to assume a nonruminant species constitutes an MAP reservoir based solely upon MAP PCR-positive findings in predators that are free of clinical disease, lack pathologic lesions, and produce culture-negative tissue cultures.

Thus, evidence of a true reservoir of MAP infection in a nonruminant population (rabbit) has been demonstrated in one locale. No other report documenting such an extensive "spill-over" of MAP infection from ruminants into other rabbit (or different lagomorph or any other nonruminant species) populations has yet appeared.

SUMMARY

All ruminant species, exotic or domestic, captive or free-ranging, are susceptible to disease and death subsequent to infection by MAP. All ruminant host species are also believed susceptible to infection by every strain of MAP so far identified; interspecies infection has been documented. Young ruminants are the most prone to infection through fecal-oral transmission: swallowing milk, colostrum, water, forage, or feed contaminated with the pathogen. Invariably fatal, Johne's disease cases have occurred in numerous zoologic hoofstock collections and thus MAP infection is of concern for an industry focused on conserving rare individual animals and their genetics. Based on studies to date, MAP may be identified (via PCR) or even isolated (via culture) from nonruminant wildlife tissues but few of these species seem to progress to organism shedding and/or disease. True nonruminant wildlife reservoirs (ie, a population capable of sustaining the infection independently of reinfection from the initial source and transmitting the pathogen to other species) are rare.

REFERENCES

1. Dargatz DA, Byrum BA, Hennager SG, et al. Prevalence of antibodies against *Mycobacterium avium* subsp. *paratuberculosis* among beef cow-calf herds. J Am Vet Med Assoc 2001;219(4):497–501.

2. Mackintosh CG, Griffin JF. Paratuberculosis in deer, camelids and other ruminants. In: Behr MA, Collins DM. eds., Paratuberculosis Organism, Disease, Control. 2010. pp. 179–87.
3. Manning EJB, Collins MT. Paratuberculosis in zoo animals. In ME Fowler and RE, Miller (eds.). Zoo & Wild Animal Medicine. Current Therapy. W.B. Saunders. Philadelphia. 1999. P. 612–6.
4. Corn JL, Manning EJ, Sreevatsan S, et al. Isolation of Mycobacterium avium subsp. paratuberculosis from free-ranging birds and mammals on livestock premises. Appl Environ Microbiol 2005;71:6963–7.
5. Manning EJB, Ziccardi M. Johne's disease and captive hoofstock: prevalence and prevention. In: Proceedings for the American Association of Zoo Veterinarians. AAZV, Media, PA. 2000. pp. 432–4
6. Witte CL, Hungerford LL, Rideout BA. Association between Mycobacterium avium subsp. paratuberculosis infection among offspring and their dams in nondomestic ruminant species housed in a zoo. J Vet Diagn Investig 2009;21:40–7.
7. Proceedings of the Workshop on Diagnosis, Prevention, and Control of Johne's Disease in Non-Domestic Hoofstock White Oak Conservation Center, Yulee, Florida. June 26-28, 1998. 1–17.
8. Stevenson K, Alvarez J, Bakker D, et al. Occurrence of Mycobacterium avium subspecies paratuberculosis across host species and European countries with evidence for transmission between wildlife and domestic ruminants. BMC Microbiol 2009.
9. Manning EJB, Kucera TE, Gates NB, et al. Testing for Mycobacterium avium subsp. paratuberculosis infection in asymptomatic free-ranging tule elk from an infected herd. J Wildl Dis 2003;39:323–8.
10. Quist CF, Nettles VF, Manning EJ, et al. Paratuberculosis in key deer (Odocoilecus virginianus clavium). J Wildl Dis 2002;38:729–37.
11. Buergelt CD, Layton AW, Ginn PE, et al. The pathology of spontaneous paratuberculosis in the North American bison (Bison bison). Vet Pathol 2000;37:428–38.
12. Corn JL, Cartwright ME, Alexy KJ, et al. Surveys for disease agents in introduced elk in Arkansas and Kentucky. J Wildl Dis 2010;46:186–94.
13. Rhyan JC, Aune K, Ewalt DR, et al. Survey of free-ranging elk from Wyoming and Montana for selected pathogens. J Wildl Dis 1997;33:290–8.
14. Davidson WR, Manning EJB, Nettles VF. Culture and serologic survey for Mycobacterium avium subsp paratuberculosis infection among Southeastern white-tailed deer (Odocoileus virginianus). J Wildl Dis 2004;40:301–6.
15. Sleeman JM, Manning EJB, Rohm JH, et al. Johne's disease in a free-ranging white-tailed deer from Virginia and subsequent surveillance for Mycobacterium avium subspecies paratuberculosis. J Wildl Dis 2009;45:201–6.
16. Pedersen K, Manning EJ, Corn JL. Distribution of Mycobacterium avium subspecies paratuberculosis in the Lower Florida Keys. J Wildl Dis 2008;44:84.
17. Kopecna M, Trcka I, Lamka J, et al. The wildlife hosts of Mycobacterium avium subsp. paratuberculosis in the Czech Republic during the years 2002-2007. Vet Med 2008;53:420–6.
18. Salgado M, Herthnek D, Bölske G, et al. First isolation of Mycobacterium avium subsp. paratuberculosis from wild guanacos (Lama guanicoe) on Tierra del Fuego Island. J of Wildl Dis 2009;45:295–301.
19. Whittington RJ, Marsh IB, Reddacliff LA. Survival of Mycobacterium avium subsp. paratuberculosis in dam water and sediment. Appl Environ Microbiol 2005;71:5304–8.

20. Hines ME, Stabel JR, Sweeney RW, et al. Experimental challenge models for Johne's disease: a review and proposed international guidelines. Vet Microbiol 2007;122: 197–222.
21. Beard P, Daniels MJ, Henderson D, et al. Paratuberculosis infection of nonruminant wildlife in Scotland. J Clin Microbiol 2001;39:1517–21.
22. Judge J, Kyriazakis I, Greig A, et al. 2005. Clustering of *Mycobacterium avium* subsp. *paratuberculosis* in rabbits and the environment: how hot is a hot spot? Appl Environ Microbiol 2005;71:6033–8.

Food Safety Concerns Regarding Paratuberculosis

Michael T. Collins, DVM, PhD

KEYWORDS

- Johne's disease • Paratuberculosis • Control
- *Mycobacterium avium* subsp. *paratuberculosis* • Food safety
- Crohn's disease

Concern about the possibility that *Mycobacterium avium* subsp. *paratuberculosis* (MAP) is a food-borne zoonotic pathogen has been the unspoken driving force behind establishment of national paratuberculosis control and herd certification programs in multiple countries including Australia, the Netherlands, Denmark, and the United States. It has also been a prime factor motivating large-scale funding of research programs like the Johne's Disease Integrated Program (JDIP) in the United States (more than US$8 million) and ParaTB Tools in the European Union (more than US$5 million). Some experts may disagree, but the true cost of paratuberculosis as a strictly animal health problem, in comparison with other infectious diseases and challenges in animal agriculture, cannot justify this magnitude of public expenditures for Johne's disease (JD) control and research unless one factors in the potential cost of paratuberculosis as a food-borne zoonotic pathogen.

IS MAP ZOONOTIC?

A wide array of animal species, including nonhuman primates, can be infected by MAP, making it quite plausible that it can also infect humans. MAP is consistently detected by PCR in humans with a disease epidemiologically and pathologically similar to JD, namely Crohn's disease (CD).[1,2] Multiple studies also detect antibody to MAP in humans with CD more often than controls. CD has been effectively treated, possibly even cured, by prolonged use of an appropriate combination of antimicrobial drugs.[3] The only significant piece of missing evidence preventing wider-spread recognition of MAP as one of the causes of CD is the inability of laboratories skilled in MAP culture to regularly grow MAP from CD patient samples.[4] That said, some laboratories have reported MAP recovery from 40 to 100% of CD patients.[5–7] MAP has also tentatively been linked with other human diseases such as type 1 diabetes mellitus.[8,9] While medical science may take more time to decide on the human health

---

The author is a paid consultant to IDEXX Laboratories, Inc.
Department of Pathobiological Sciences, School of Veterinary Medicine, University of Wisconsin, 2015 Linden Drive, Madison, WI 53706-1102, USA
E-mail address: mcollin5@wisc.edu

Vet Clin Food Anim 27 (2011) 631–636
doi:10.1016/j.cvfa.2011.07.009 **vetfood.theclinics.com**

consequences of MAP exposure, it is prudent for veterinary medicine to consider what can be done to mitigate the risk of human exposure to this potentially zoonotic ruminant pathogen.

RAW FOOD CONTAMINATION BY MAP

The majority of MAP infections occur in food-producing ruminants (ie, cattle, goats, and sheep) (see article by Lombard in this issue). Meat and milk derived from MAP-infected animals is commonly contaminated before harvesting (ie, ante mortem) during the disseminated stage of MAP infections when the organism is found in muscle meat, internal organs, colostrum and milk, and the unborn fetus of pregnant animals[10–12] (see the article by Sweeney in this issue). During harvesting of both milk and meat, there is a second opportunity for MAP contamination of food products in conjunction with fecal contamination.[13] Thus, raw products originating from herds or flocks of MAP-infected animals are likely to be contaminated with MAP.[14] Counts up to 560 MAP/mL of raw milk from individual cows have been reported.[13] The question then becomes whether manufacturing processes or cooking by the consumer will reliably kill MAP.

PASTEURIZED FOOD PRODUCTS

The preponderance of work on the ability of food manufacturing processes to kill MAP has focused on pasteurization, specifically high-temperature short-time (HTST) pasteurization.[15] Laboratory studies attempting to measure standard thermal tolerance parameters for MAP indicate that it is more heat-resistant than *Mycobacterium bovis* and *Coxiella burnetti*, the 2 milk-borne zoonotic pathogens designed to be killed by pasteurization.[16,17] Corroborating this are 3 independent retail milk surveys reporting recovery of viable MAP by culture from retail HTST pasteurized milk.[18–20] Clearly, HTST pasteurization kills large numbers of MAP in milk. However, evidence suggests that it does not kill 100% of MAP cells 100% of the time or that postpasteurization MAP contamination is frequently occurring.

Cheese

High-moisture, high-pH, "fresh" (short time from production to consumption) cheeses made from raw milk have the greatest likelihood of containing MAP as well as other milk-borne bacterial pathogens like *Listeria*.[21] However, MAP has been shown to persist even the processes involved in making low-moisture, low pH, aged cheese such as Swiss cheese, regardless of whether milk was first pasteurized.[22,23]

Yoghurt and Other Dairy Products

MAP numbers in spiked yoghurt were shown to persist during storage but decline somewhat in the presence of certain probiotic bacteria found in fermented milk products.[24] Other dairy products such as ice cream or powdered milk preparations have not been studied.

Meat

The effect of cooking on MAP viability in meat has been studied far less than pasteurization. Empirically, if meat is cooked to a condition known as "well-done" (defined as when the meat juices run clear), then the center of the product has attained a core temperature equivalent to that of HTST pasteurization. Hence, one could predict low or no MAP recovery from well-done meat. This prediction is supported by 2 studies attempting recovery of MAP from naturally and intentionally contaminated meat.[25,26] Meat that is not well-done could harbor viable MAP.

Ground beef represents the greatest potential risk for harboring MAP in that (1) a significant proportion originates from culled dairy cattle, which have the highest animal-level prevalence of MAP infections; (2) dairy cattle are culled when they are no longer productive and late-stage MAP infections are a cause of low productivity; (3) fecal contamination of carcasses in the abattoir occurs despite efforts to minimize it; (4) ground beef includes lymph nodes where MAP are concentrated; and (5) the process of mixing and grinding beef to produce hamburger blends any MAP into the final product, away from the surface, which is exposed to the highest level of heat during cooking. However, the frequency of finding viable MAP in retail meat has not been assessed. Arguably, *Escherichia coli* O157 may serve as an indicator organism to gauge the frequency with which a zoonotic bacterial pathogen found in cattle feces contaminates ground beef. If one accepts this premise, then the frequent ground beef recalls due to *E. coli* O157 detection in the United States suggests that MAP contamination of ground beef may be common (Available at: http://www.fsis.usda.gov/Fsis_recalls/Open_Federal_Cases/index.asp; Accessed March 24, 2011).

Water

Although not traditionally considered "food," domestic water supplies must be considered in the context of food safety to ensure a balanced perspective on potential modes of human exposure to MAP. Domestic water sources vary among and within communities. Tap water may originate from surface water (ie, lakes and rivers) or underground (ie, wells). Surface waters are generally a mix of rainwater runoff and artesian spring water. Rainwater falling on land occupied by MAP-infected cattle has the potential to harbor MAP and the organism will persist in rainwater runoff for a prolonged time (eg, >1 year).[27] *Mycobacteria,* including MAP, are resistant to killing by the levels of chlorine commonly used to decontaminate domestic water.[28,29] Hence, water may exposure humans to MAP via either drinking or aerosolization and inhalation.[30–32]

SUMMARY

Two recent risk assessments concur in the conclusion that MAP contaminates raw products derived from MAP-infected animals and water runoff from MAP-infected farms and that MAP may survive food manufacturing processes or cooking.[33,34] The provocative discovery that MAP can produce spores explains its persistence in the environment and its tenacity in the face of industrial processes designed to control food-borne bacterial pathogens.[35] It remains to be proved what the real health consequences of MAP exposure or infection are for humans, and it will take considerable time and effort for medical science to resolve this question due, in part, to the chronic insidious nature of the diseases potentially involved and the lack of well-standardized assays for MAP infection in humans. However, given the weight of evidence and the severity and magnitude of potential human health problems, the precautionary principle suggests that it is time to take actions to limit "as low as reasonably achievable" human exposure to MAP.[36] All evidence suggests that the farm is the critical control point. Paratuberculosis control on farms serves to improve animal health and welfare, improve farm profitability, and lower MAP numbers in raw food products, thereby lessening the likelihood and level of human exposure to MAP whether in dairy products, meat, or domestic water supplies. With the rapid globalization of food production and trade, the challenge of MAP control for both animal health and consumer confidence in the safety of their food is international.

REFERENCES

1. Abubakar I, Myhill D, Aliyu SH, et al. Detection of *Mycobacterium avium* subspecies *paratuberculosis* from patients with Crohn's disease using nucleic acid-based techniques: a systematic review and meta-analysis. Inflamm Bowel Dis 2008; 14(3):401–10.
2. Feller M, Huwiler K, Stephan R, et al. *Mycobacterium avium* subspecies *paratuberculosis* and Crohn's disease: a systematic review and meta-analysis. Lancet Infect Dis 2007;7(9):607–13.
3. Chamberlin W, Ghobrial G, Chehtane M, et al. Successful treatment of a Crohn's disease patient infected with bacteremic *Mycobacterium paratuberculosis*. Am J Gastroenterol 2007;102(3):689–91.
4. Behr MA. Paratuberculosis and Crohn's disease. In: Behr MA, Collins DM, editors. Paratuberculosis: organism,disease, control. Oxfordshlre, UK: CABI; 2010. p. 40–9.
5. Mendoza JL, San-Pedro A, Culebras E, et al. High prevalence of vaible *Mycobacterium avium* subspecies *paratuberculosis* in Crohn's disease. World J Gastroenterol 2010;16(36):4558–63.
6. Naser SA, Collins MT, Crawford JT, et al. Culture of *Mycobacterium avium* subspecies *paratuberculosis* (MAP) from the blood of patients with Crohn's disease: A follow-up blind multi-center investigation. Open Inflamm J 2009;222-3.
7. Naser SA, Ghobrial G, Romero C, et al. Culture of *Mycobacterium avium* subspecies *paratuberculosis* from the blood of patients with Crohn's disease. Lancet 2004;364:1039–44.
8. Dow CT. Paratuberculosis and Type I diabetes: is this the trigger? Med Hypoth 2006;67(4):782–5.
9. Sechi LA, Rosu V, Pacifico A, et al. Humoral immune responses of Type 1 Diabetes patients to *Mycobacterium avium* subsp. *paratuberculosis* lend support to the infectious trigger hypothesis. Clin Vaccine Immunol 2008;15(2):320–6.
10. Alonso-Hearn M, Molina E, Geijo M, et al. Isolation of *Mycobacterium avium* subsp. *paratuberculosis* from muscle tissue of naturally infected cattle. Foodborne Pathogens Dis 2009;6(4):513–8.
11. Antognoli MC, Garry FB, Hirst HL, et al. Characterization of *Mycobacterium avium* subspecies *paratuberculosis* dissemination in dairy cattle and its association with antemortem test results. Vet Microbiol 2008;127;300–8.
12. Brady C, O'Grady D, O'Meara F, et al. Relationships between clinical signs, pathological changes and tissue distribution of *Mycobacterium avium* subspecies *paratuberculosis* in 21 cows from herds affected by Johne's disease. Vet Rec 2008;162(5): 147–52.
13. Grant IR. *Mycobacterium avium* subsp. *paratuberculosis* in animal-derived foods and the environment. In: Behr MA, Collins DM, editors. Paratuberculosis: organism,disease, control. Oxfordshire, UK: CABI; 2010. p. 29–39.
14. Eltholth MM, Marsh VR, Van Winden S, et al. Contamination of food products with *Mycobacterium avium paratuberculosis*: a systematic review. J Appl Microbiol 2009; 107;1061–71.
15. Grant IR, Hitchings EI, McCartney A, et al. Effect of commercial-scale high-temperature, short-time pasteurization on the viability of *Mycobacterium paratuberculosis* in naturally infected cows' milk. Appl Env Microbiol 2002;68(2):602–7.

16. Stumbo CR. Organisms of greatest importance in food pasteurization. In: Thermo-bacteriology in food processing. 2nd edition. New York: Academic Press; 1973. p. 31–45.
17. Sung N, Collins MT. Thermal tolerance of *Mycobacterium paratuberculosis*. Appl Env Microbiol 1998;64;999–1005.
18. Ayele WY, Svastova P, Roubal P, et al. *Mycobacterium avium* subspecies *paratuberculosis* cultured from locally and commercially pasteurized cow's milk in the Czech Republic. Appl Env Microbiol 2005;71;1210–4.
19. Ellingson JLE, Anderson JL, Koziczkowski JJ, et al. Detection of viable *Mycobacterium avium* subsp. *paratuberculosis* in retail pasteurized whole milk by two culture methods and PCR. J Food Prot 2005;67;966–72.
20. Grant IR, Ball HJ, Rowe MT. Incidence of *Mycobacterium paratuberculosis* in bulk raw and commercially pasteurized cows' milk from approved dairy processing establishments in the United Kingdom. Appl Env Microbiol 2002;682;428–35.
21. Sung N, Collins MT. Effect of three factors in cheese production (pH, salt, and heat) on *Mycobacterium avium* subsp *paratuberculosis* viability. Appl Env Microbiol 2000; 66(4):1334–9.
22. Spahr U, Schafroth K. Fate of *Mycobacterium avium* subsp *paratuberculosis* in Swiss hard and semihard cheese manufactured from raw milk. Appl Env Microbiol 2001; 67(9):4199–205.
23. Williams AG, Withers SE. Microbiological characterisation of artisanal farmhouse cheeses manufacturered in Scotland. Int J Dairy Technol 2010;63(3):356–69.
24. Van Brandt L, Coudijzer K, Herman L, et al. Survival of *Mycobacterium avium* ssp. *paratuberculosis* in yoghurt and in commercial fermented milk products containing probiotic cultures. J Appl Microbiol 2011;110(5):1252–61.
25. Mutharia LM, Klassen MD, Fairles J, et al. *Mycobacterium avium* subsp. *paratuberculosis* in muscle, lymphatic and organ tissues from cows with advanced Johne's disease. Int J Food Microbiol 2010;136(3):340–4.
26. Whittington RJ, Waldron A, Warne D. Thermal inactivation profiles of *Mycobacterium avium* subsp. *paratuberculosis* in lamb skeletal muscle homogenate fluid. Int J Food Microbiol 2009.
27. Whittington RJ, Marsh IB, Reddacliff LA. Survival of *Mycobacterium avium* subsp. *paratuberculosis* in dam water and sediment. Appl Env Microbiol 2005;71(9):5304–8.
28. Le Dantec C, Duguet JP, Montiel A, et al. Chlorine disinfection of atypical mycobacteria isolated from a water distribution system. Appl Env Microbiol 2002;68(3):1025–32.
29. Whan LB, Grant IR, Ball HJ, et al. Bactericidal effect of chlorine on *Mycobacterium paratuberculosis* in drinking water. Lett Appl Microbiol 2001;33(3):227–31.
30. Beumer A, King D, Donohue M, et al. Detection of *Mycobacterium avium* subsp. *paratuberculosis* in drinking water and biofilms by quantitative PCR. Appl Env Microbiol 2010;76(21):7367–70.
31. Falkingham JO III. Nontuberculous mycobacteria from household plumbing of patients with nontuberculous mycobacteria disease. Emerg Infect Dis 2011;17(3): 419-4.
32. Pickup RW, Rhodes G, Arnott S, et al. *Mycobacterium avium* subspecies *paratuberculosis* in the catchment and water of the river Taff in South Wales, UK and its potential relationship to clustering of Crohn's disease in the city of Cardiff. Appl Env Microbiol 2005;71(4):2130–9.
33. Gill CO, Saucier L, Meadus WJ. *Mycobacterium avium* subsp. *paratuberculosis* in dairy products, meat, and drinking water. J Food Prot 2011;74(3):480–99.

34. National Advisory Committee on Microbiological Criteria for Foods. Assessment of food as a source of exposure to *Mycobacterium avium* subspecies *paratuberculosis* (MAP). J Food Prot 2010;73(7):1357–97.

35. Lamont EA, Bannantine JP, Armien A, et al. *Mycobacterium avium* subspecies *paratuberculosis* produces spores. Presented at the 110th Annual General Meeting of American Society of Microbiology. San Diego, CA, 2010 [abstract: U2932].

36. Weir E, Schabas R, Wilson K, et al. A Canadian framework for applying the precautionary principle to public health issues. Can J Pub Health 2010;101(5):396–8.

State, Federal, and Industry Efforts at Paratuberculosis Control

Michael A. Carter, DVM, MPH

KEYWORDS
- Paratuberculosis • Federal • State • Control • Certification

In 1996, the US Department of Agriculture's (USDA) Animal and Plant Health Inspection Service (APHIS), Veterinary Services (VS), National Animal Health Monitoring System (NAHMS) conducted a national dairy study to evaluate various aspects of dairy on-farm management. One objective of this study was the first attempt at estimating the national herd prevalence for Johne's disease (JD).[1] The study provided a conservative estimate of 22% herd prevalence and found that fewer than 1% of dairy herds participated in a JD herd certification program. The study also showed that approximately 45% of dairy producers knew nothing or very little about JD.[1] A similar study was completed for beef cattle in 1997, which estimated the herd prevalence for JD at 7.9%, with 92.2% of beef producers knowing nothing or very little about the disease.[2]

A follow-up NAHMS dairy study conducted in 2007 increased the estimated national herd prevalence to 68.1%.[3] While the prevalence numbers appear to be increasing, and only 10% of dairy producers are officially enrolled in the Voluntary Bovine Johne's Disease Control Program (the national program adopted by APHIS), the study reported that 31.7% of the producers participated in a JD control program of some kind and 35.3% tested for JD in their herds.[4] These study results are disappointing; however, the numbers suggest that APHIS' greatest positive impact on the control of JD may be providing education and training opportunities to cattle producers.

HISTORY OF JOHNE'S CONTROL IN THE UNITED STATES
National Regulations

The USDA has a long history of regulatory control of paratuberculosis. As early as 1952, the Secretary of Agriculture issued a notice that paratuberculosis existed in

The author has nothing to disclose.

Ruminant Health Programs, National Center for Animal Health Programs, Veterinary Services, Animal and Plant Health Inspection Service, US Department of Agriculture, 4700 River Road, Unit 43, Riverdale, MD 20737, USA

E-mail address: michael.a.carter@aphia.usda.gov

Vet Clin Food Anim 27 (2011) 637–645
doi:10.1016/j.cvfa.2011.07.010
0749-0720/11/$ – see front matter Published by Elsevier Inc.

Puerto Rico and in each state of the continental United States, except Maine, New Hampshire, Rhode Island, Utah, and Wyoming.[5] Since then, various regulations have been implemented to control the national spread of JD, but none have been effective; JD is now considered to exist in all areas of the United States.

In April 2000, APHIS changed its JD regulations to restrict animal movement only after they have been confirmed positive by an official JD test (defined as an organism detection test conducted in a USDA-approved laboratory). These animals are restricted to the state-of-origin unless they are sent directly to slaughter.[6] If the animals are sent to slaughter, an owner/shipper statement identifying the animals as infected is required. One weakness of this regulation is that animals suspected of having JD typically may be culled due to clinical disease or other management reasons without confirmatory testing or before the results from the official JD tests are received by the veterinarian or producer. This delay could potentially allow animals that are shedding the organism to enter back into live animal markets. The reason for not restricting movements for any animal with a test-positive result was to encourage producers to incorporate testing as a strategy for on-farm management of the disease. With current heavy reliance on serum and milk enzyme-linked immunosorbent assay (ELISA) tests, farm owners can test and remove animals from the premises with minimal regulatory restrictions.

Voluntary Certification Programs

In 1993, US Animal Health Association adopted a model JD herd certification program.[7] This program was not readily accepted by the industry because of program issues and associated costs for testing all animals above 24 months of age in a herd. In an effort to develop a program that would be more appealing to cattle producers, USAHA's National Johne's Working Group (NJWG) appointed a committee of federal, state, and industry representatives to design a more affordable and flexible program based on current scientific knowledge. The result was the U.S. Voluntary Johne's Disease Herd Status Program for Cattle (VJDHSP).[8] The focus of the program was to identify herds with a low risk for the presence of *Mycobacterium avium* subsp. *paratuberculosis* (MAP) infection, instead of certifying herds as free (which requires more intensive testing). The VJDHSP guidelines were used by states in developing JD control programs. This led to the creation of the Uniform Program Standards for the Voluntary Bovine Johne's Disease Control Program (VBJDCP) by industry, state, and federal personnel. The first version of the new VBJDCP was approved by APHIS in April 2002.[9]

The objective of the VBJDCP is to provide minimal national standards for the classification of herds with low risk of having JD and to provide an organized approach to controlling the disease at the producer level. Although the VBJDCP does not preclude the adoption of more stringent rules by any state with regard to activities within its boundaries, it is hoped that states will make only minor changes to how the program is administered.

In 2010, APHIS revised the program standards to decrease the complexity of the certification program and to allow more flexibility in the testing options available to producers. The new program standards eliminated the separate test-negative and test-positive components and adopted a gradient approach to herd classification.[10]

National Funding

APHIS has dedicated funding and resources to a national JD control effort since fiscal year (FY) 2000. FY 2003 was the first year that the U.S. Congress included a specific line item in USDA's budget for the JD program and was also the high point of congressional funding for the program with $21 million allocated for control activities. Since 2000, Congress (through USDA-APHIS) has committed more than $118 million to the national effort, with $48 million of that funding distributed directly to states and universities in the form of cooperative agreements to aid producers at the state level. In 2003 and 2004, large portions of the funding went toward improving state and laboratory capacity to deal with the increased program management and testing needs that resulted from JD education campaigns.

States have used their own resources to educate producers and veterinarians to build awareness, and funds received by states through federal cooperative agreements with USDA have been used to provide incentives for producers to join the VBJDCP. These incentives include testing cost supplementation and covering the veterinary fees for conducting risk assessments and developing herd management plans. Two states (New York and Wisconsin) have attempted to provide small grants to producers to encourage management changes. Although these grants were appreciated by producers, they also placed significant burdens on state administrations to review, approve, and monitor the grants. These administrative burdens subsequently resulted in the programs continuing for only a few years.

CURRENT NATIONAL PROGRAM

The VBJDCP is a cooperative program administered by state animal health agencies and supported by industry and federal agencies. The program consists of 3 basic elements: (1) education, (2) management, and (3) herd testing and classification.

Most states have adopted the national program as is, while others have included the VBJDCP as part of a larger quality assurance/cattle health program, providing a broader approach to disease prevention and management issues on premises. This format is a practical approach for the voluntary program, particularly as federal funding continues to decrease.

Education Effort

The education component of the program is intended to inform livestock producers about the costs of JD (from the loss of production and disease management) and to provide information about management strategies to prevent, control, and eliminate the disease. Each state has developed its own approach to implementing this aspect of the program. In some states, the effort may be as simple as contacting producers after a positive test result is reported or offering periodic seminars for producers and veterinarians. Examples of university-led online efforts may be viewed at *http://www.johnes.org site* (University of Wisconsin) for producers and industry, *http://vetmdce.org site* (University of Wisconsin Veterinary School of Veterinary Medicine) for veterinary continuing education, and *http://nyschap.vet.cornell.edu/ site* (Cornell University; includes a JD module) for participants of the New York Cattle Health Assurance Program.

To provide information at a national level, USDA funds 3 major projects to collect and disseminate information related to the diagnosis, control, and management of JD: the National Johne's Disease Demonstration Herd Project, the National Johne's Education Initiative, and the Johne's Disease Integrated Program.

National Johne's Disease Demonstration Herd Project

The National Johne's Disease Demonstration Herd Project (NJDDHP) was proposed in 2002 and was officially implemented in 2003 through funding from APHIS; although several states had initiated their own state-funded projects previous to 2003. The primary objective of the demonstration herd project was to evaluate the long-term effectiveness and feasibility of management-related disease control measures for JD. Secondary objectives included providing information for education and training, evaluating management, testing and monitoring strategies, and creating well-characterized herds to address other research objectives.[11] To accomplish this, the project captured specific outcomes for each herd in the project for analysis. Examples of these outcomes include the incidence of clinical disease and prevalence of infection, the amount of culling done based on test results, and the evaluation and monitoring of disease-transmission risks resulting from on-farm management practices.

The NJDDHP completed its data collection in September 2010. Sixteen states with dairy herds participated and 11 states enrolled beef herds. Twenty-three beef herds and 66 dairy herds completed the project, accounting for approximately 6400 and 74,000 mature cattle (2 years or older), respectively. Approximately 116,000 animals were sampled and an estimated 460,000 tests were conducted during the course of the 7-year project. Participating beef herds ranged from 35 to more than 700 mature cattle; while dairy operations ranged in size from 70 to more than 4000 lactating cows (Charles Fossler, Fort Collins, CO, personal communication, August 12, 2010).

The largest percentage of both beef and dairy herds consisted of herds ranging from 100 to 499 mature cattle. The project resulted in 25 peer review papers in addition to lay articles and industry group presentations given around the country. Additional written products are expected to be produced as the data analysis continues through 2011.

National Johne's Education Initiative

The National Johne's Education Initiative (NJEI) was developed in response to the needs identified in the 2002 National Johne's Disease Control Program Strategic Plan.[12] The initiative focuses on producer outreach and is a collaboration between APHIS and the National Institute of Animal Agriculture, with contributions from states, universities, and industry groups. The goal of NJEI is to enhance awareness of JD within the livestock community, thereby increasing producers' implementation of best management practices to target JD transmission and to increase participation in the VBJDCP. Activities of the NJEI include drafting educational articles for inclusion in leading producer publications, developing and distributing press releases when new information becomes available, creating and distributing brochures, factsheets, and newsletters, and maintaining a website (www.johnesdisease.org) to distribute information and direct information seekers to other useful sites from a central access point.[13]

Johne's Disease Integrated Program

The Johne's Disease Integrated Program (JDIP) is an association of scientists from various universities to promote animal biosecurity to reduce the risk of JD transmission within and among herds.[14] JDIP's activities are funded primarily through a Cooperative State Research, Education, and Extension Service-National Research Institute grant (now the National Institute of Food and Agriculture) from USDA. The primary goal of JDIP is to promote efficient biosecurity practices on-farm through collaborative research and to share resources that are critical to the success of the JD research community. In addition to the core resources and funding outside of developmental projects, four collaborative research projects have been developed to meet the needs of the stakeholders. The projects focus on epidemiology and transmission; diagnostics and strain differentiation; biology and pathogenesis; and immunology and vaccine development. Information developed as a result of JDIP's efforts is disseminated through JDIP's outreach group which translates the scientific information into material for producer publications. The end goal of JDIP is to reduce the time between basic scientific research and the development of useful products and procedures.

Disease Management

The management component of the program provides a systematic evaluation of producers' operations and a framework to develop herd management plans that address risky practices that could allow the transmission of MAP among animals or between premises. Using manuals to guide the process, the program provides best management practices that, when implemented, reduce the risk of transmission. A risk assessment conducted by veterinarians trained to use JD program material helps to identify specific risky practices for use by producers to target changes on their premises.

In addition to management changes, vaccination is a control tool used in the program because it reduces the clinical signs of JD. However, the current licensed vaccine product does not prevent infection.[15] Due to the ability of MAP to cause cross-reactions on tests for other mycobacteria, widespread vaccination is not encouraged by APHIS because vaccinated animals could cause an increase in false-positive responses to the caudal fold test for tuberculosis. This increase could have an impact when targeting beef cattle, but it may not have a significant impact in the reaction rate in dairy cattle because of the high endemic rate of JD. Further evaluation of the impact of JD vaccination is needed.

A second tool is testing to identify potential carriers of MAP. The classification component of the program dictates the amount and type of testing herd owners are required to conduct, but the education and management component of the VBJDCP does not specify testing protocols. Herd owners that are involved only with the education level of the program typically have not done any testing because the education component is usually the first contact that these producers have had with the program. Herd owners participating at the management component are not required to test, but most owners incorporate some kind of testing in their herd management plans. The testing is intended to be a "best fit" according to the needs and resources of producers and can be quite flexible. To assist producers and veterinarians with identifying an appropriate testing strategy, APHIS supported a project to develop a "Best Test Strategies" document. The final report was published in 2006 and provided a simplified set of recommendations for veterinarians and producers that were categorized by cattle type (beef or dairy) and by the goal of the testing. Examples of possible testing goals include estimates of biological burden, eradication, control, and disease confirmation.[16]

Herd Classification

The VBJDCP included a herd classification component to the program in 2002 to facilitate the identification of test-negative herds to provide producers additional information regarding the level of confidence with the low risk status or an estimated prevalence within infected herds.[9] This classification component used the guidance outlined by the VJDHSP and recommendations from "Minimum Recommendations for Administering and Instituting State Voluntary Johne's Disease Programs for Cattle."[17] The program component was based on the knowledge that a single herd test would not be adequate to detect 100% of the infected herds, but with multiple years of testing, most infected herds could be detected.

In 2010, APHIS revised the program standards to decrease the complexity of the certification program and to allow greater flexibility in testing options available to producers. The new program standards eliminated separate test-negative and test-positive components and adopted a gradient approach to the levels.[10] This approach classifies herds based on a 95% confidence that herds within a given level would be less than a specified prevalence (15% for level 1, 10% for level 2, 5% for level 3, and 2% for level 4 and greater).[18] Based on assumptions for test sensitivity and specificity, a table was created to estimate the true prevalence range based on the test used and the number of test-eligible animals, and used that estimate to classify the herd. This revised classification method will allow a more rapid inclusion of new test methods after the test diagnostic sensitivity and specificity are estimated and validated.

STATE EFFORTS

While the program remains voluntary at the state and producer level, the VBJDCP provides the standard for which all state programs are operated in order to provide a level of consistency between states. To make the best use of state infrastructure and to match the needs of the cattle industry of the state, various states have implemented the program in different ways. The most active states (in terms of testing and enrolled herds) are Minnesota, New York, Ohio, Pennsylvania, and Wisconsin.

Minnesota was an early adopter of the VJDHSP. When APHIS approved the 2002 Uniform Program Standards for the VBJDCP, Minnesota animal health authorities were already preparing to adopt the new standards, and for much of the program's existence, the state had the greatest number of herds enrolled. Minnesota's approach was to adopt the program as written in the program standards to start their Johne's Disease Control Program. Because it is a voluntary program, Minnesota did not need to change any regulations to meet the program requirements, thereby allowing immediate program implementation. As of May of 2009, Minnesota has tested more than 435,130 cattle in approximately 5606 herds.[19]

The New York State Cattle Health Assurance Program is a state-funded program built on a core of best management practices such as animal identification, record-keeping, and general health. The state program has added additional modules to the core requirements, including JD or *Salmonella* control, animal welfare, and environmental protection. Participants must complete the core requirements; but producers may choose which modules, if any, fit the needs of individual premises. Most enrolled premises participated in the JD module because of enrollment benefits from subsidized testing costs. [20]

Ohio adopted the earlier JD herd certification model and continued to use that approach during the early years of the VBJDCP. Due to the cost of the testing portion of the program, the State subsidized the testing costs to ease the burden on producers.

Pennsylvania also modeled their program after the VBJDCP, and similar to Minnesota, the state has not significantly altered the way the program is operated nor does it require the codification of the program rules. All of the components of the VBJDCP are present in Pennsylvania; however, the state has a clear segregation of the management level of the program from the herd certification program.[21]

Wisconsin developed and implemented a 4-stage classification program as a way to limit producer liability when selling cattle prior to APHIS' adoption of the VBJDCP. This state program was based on test prevalence rates beginning with level D (a herd test prevalence >15%) to level A (in which herds had no test positive animals).[22] This A, B, C, D classification system was blended with the VJDHSP to create the VBJDCP as adopted by APHIS. Wisconsin has used the VBJDCP since 2002, although more emphasis was on the A–D classification as a result of their regulations in the early years. Unlike Minnesota, and despite voluntary participation in the VBJDCP, the program rules must be codified in Wisconsin in order to be official. This process delays implementation after rules change at the national level (other states also fall into this category). From October 2003 until October 2010, Wisconsin has reported testing more than 1,388,000 samples (National Johne's disease quarterly reports, November 2010).

It must be noted that the 5 states discussed above had JD control programs in place before the adoption of the federally approved VBJDCP; the only current difference is increased consistency. Also, all of these states have invested state funds into program activities and producer incentives. These 2 factors seem to have the greatest impact on how eagerly producers adopted the new program.

INDUSTRY INITIATIVES

Industry remains a key partner in outreach effort to producers. Beef organizations have been providing Johne's information to members but had limited interaction with state activities. For the dairy industry, organizations such as cooperatives and producer and breed associations function primarily as a conduit for information to their members. The current economic downturn had caused several organizations to focus their efforts on short-term economic issues rather than targeting longer-term animal health issues. Organic Valley is an example of one cooperator that is working aggressively with members to increase JD awareness by providing bulk tank screening tests, reduced prices for milk ELISA testing, and actively encouraging risk assessments and management plans on member farms.[23]

The involvement of the Dairy Herd Improvement Association (DHIA) system continues to evolve. DHIA service units act as a conduit for information dissemination but is also providing milk ELISA testing services. Several of the DHIA laboratories are also approved for culture, PCR, and serum ELISA, thereby allowing the provision of various testing options for producers and veterinarians. Dairy Records Processing Centers associated with the DHIA system are becoming data repositories for JD testing results (along with other herd production data), which provides producers the ability to compare test results alongside production data.[23]

SUMMARY

Over the past decade, the cattle industry, state animal health agencies and USDA APHIS have invested significant resources for education and outreach to producers and to the control of JD. This effort has resulted in the successful development of a strong infrastructure to support the program in many states, including the critical components of laboratory capacity and trained veterinarians to conduct risk assessments and design effective management plans on cattle operations. However, the key to JD control remains at the premises level. Government programs cannot replace well-thought-out plans by producers that are specific to individual farms, resources, facilities, and management practices.

REFERENCES

1. USDA. Johne's disease on U.S. dairy operations. Fort Collins (CO): USDA-APHIS-VS-CEAH; 1997. No. N245.1097.
2. USDA. Part III: Reference of 1997 beef cow-calf production management and disease control. Fort Collins (CO): USDA-APHIS-VS-CEAH; 1998. No. N247.198.
3. USDA. Johne's disease on U.S. dairies, 1991–2007. Fort Collins (CO): USDA-APHIS-VS-CEAH; 2008. No. N521.0408.
4. USDA. Dairy 2007, part V: changes in dairy cattle health and management practices in the United States, 1996–2007. Fort Collins (CO): USDA-APHIS-VS-CEAH; 2009. No. 519.0709.

5. NARA. Department of Agriculture, Office of the Secretary, brucellosis and paratuberculosis: notice regarding contagion of communicable disease. Federal Register. Washington, DC: Office of the Federal Register, National Archives and Records Administration, vol. 17. June 9, 1952. p. 5260.

6. NARA. Animal and Plant Health Inspection Service 9 CFR 71 and 80: Johne's disease in domestic livestock; interstate movement. Federal Register. Washington, DC: Office of the Federal Register, National Archives and Records Administration, April 10, 2000. Vol. 65, No. 69, p. 18875–9.

7. Whipple D. National Paratuberculosis Certification Program. In: United States Animal Health Association Proceedings: Report of the 97th Annual Meeting of the United States Animal Health Association. Las Vegas, October 23–29, 1993, p. 311–6.

8. Bulga LL. U.S. voluntary Johne's disease herd status program for cattle. In: United States Animals Health Association Proceedings: Report of the 102nd Annual Meeting of the United Stated Animal Health Association. Minneapolis, 1998. p. 420–33.

9. USDA. Uniform program standards for the voluntary bovine Johne's Disease Control Program. Riverdale (MD): USDA-APHIS; 2002. No. 91-45-014.

10. USDA. Uniform program standards for the voluntary bovine Johne's Disease Control Program. Riverdale (MD): USDA-APHIS; 2010. No. 91-45-016.

11. USDA. National Johne's Disease Demonstration Herd Project. Fort Collins (CO): USDA-APHIS-VS-CEAH; 2005. No. N442.1005.

12. Hartman WL. Committee on Johne's Disease: Report of the Ad Hoc Steering Subcommittee. In: United States Animals Health Association Proceedings: Report of the 106th Annual Meeting of the United Stated Animal Health Association. St Louis: 2002. p. 336–41.

13. NIAA. National Johne's Disease Education Initiative. National Institute of Animal Agriculture. October 1, 2010. Available at: http://www.johnesdisease.org. Accessed July 19, 2011.

14. JDIP. Johne's Disease Integrated Program. Johne's Disease Integrated Program. October 1, 2010. Available at: http://www.jdip.org. Accessed July 19, 2011.

15. Fort Dodge Animal Health. Mycopar® Label. Fort Dodge Mycobacterium Paratuberculosis Bacterin. Fort Dodge, IA: 2007. Vol. U.S. Vet. License 112.

16. Collin MT, Gardner IA, Garry FB, et al. Consensus recommendations on diagnostic testing for the detection of paratuberculosis in cattle in the United States. J Am Vet Med Assoc 2006;229:1912–9.

17. Bulaga LL. Minimum recommendations for administering and instituting state voluntary Johne's Disease Control Programs. In: United States Animals Health Association Proceedings: Report of the 103nd Annual Meeting of the United States Animal Health Association. Minneapolis, 1999. p. 336–55.

18. Tavornpanicha S, Wells SJ, Fossler C, et al. Improved method of herd classification for the U.S. voluntary bovine Johne's Disease Control Program. Am J Vet Res, accepted for publication.

19. Minnesota Board of Animal Health. Minnesota voluntary Johne's Disease Control Program. Minnesota Board of Animal Health: Johne's Disease. May 23, 2009. Available at: http://www.bah.state.mn.us/diseases/johnes/index.html. Accessed July 19, 2011.

20. New York State Department of Agriculture and Marketing. New York State Cattle Health Assurance Program. 2002. Available at: http://nyschap.vet.cornell.edu/default.asp. Accessed July 19, 2011.

21. Pennsylvania Department of Agriculture. Johne's Disease Certification. Pennsylvania Department of Agriculture, Bureau of Animal Health and Diagnostic Services. 2010. Available at: http://www.agriculture.state.pa.us/portal/server.pt/gateway/PTARGS_0_2_24476_10297_0_43/http%3B/10.41.0.36/AgWebsite/ProgramDetail.aspx?name=Johnes-Disease-&navid=12&parentnavid=0&palid=37&. Accessed July 19, 2011.

22. Wisconsin Department of Agriculture, Trade and Consumer Protection. Johne's Disease Control Program. Wisconsin Department of Agriculture, Trade and Consumer Protection- Animal Welfare and Disease. Available at: http://datcp.state.wi.us/ah/agriculture/animals/disease/johnes/index.jsp. Accessed July 19, 2011.
23. Olson K. Johne's education and outreach efforts and impacts 2009–2010 report and development and beta test of an instrument for assessing producer use of JD management practices, Johne's Disease Integrated Program Report to USDA-APHIS-VS. JDIP: March 2010.

International Efforts at Paratuberculosis Control

David Kennedy, BVSc, MVS, MACVSc

KEYWORDS

- Paratuberculosis • Johne's • International • Control
- Assurance

Johne's disease is now playing on a truly global stage thanks to the trucks, ships, and aircraft that have moved animals around the world in the past century. In late 2010, only 26 countries were listed as reporting that the disease had never occurred in their country.[1] *Mycobacterium avium* subsp. *paratuberculosis* (MAP) slowly spread out from western Europe in live animal exports to colonies and other markets. This year is the centenary of the first confirmed case in Australia—an imported bull in a quarantine station.[2] As the livestock industries matured in countries in the Americas and Pacific, they in turn contributed to Johne's disease spreading to trading partners that had only more recently developed their domestic livestock production systems. The increased incidence of Johne's disease in eastern Europe was largely attributed to the development of the livestock trade from western Europe after the fall of the "Iron Curtain."[3] Recently, Johne's disease, caused by various subtypes of MAP, has been recognised as a developing problem in a diverse range of countries including Iran,[4] South Africa,[5] India,[6] and Korea.[7]

This progressive, inadvertent spread of MAP over long distances has been favored by 2 of its key characteristics: the largely subclinical nature of infection and the poor sensitivity of diagnostic tests. In the past 20 years, the international community has attempted to limit this spread and its impacts.

INTERNATIONAL COLLABORATION

International interest in Johne's disease increased toward the end of the twentieth century, following the publication of work by Chiodini and others associating MAP with Crohn's disease in people in the United States.[8] Multinational groups have addressed various aspects of understanding and managing paratuberculosis, much of it stimulated by ongoing debate about this hypothesis.

Founded in 1989, The International Association for Paratuberculosis is a "scientific organization devoted to the advancement of scientific progress on paratuberculosis

The author is the National Technical Adviser to Animal Health Australia's National Johne's Disease Control Program. The position is funded through levies paid by Australian livestock producers.

AusVet Animal Health Services Pty Ltd, PO Box 2321, Orange, New South Wales, 2800 Australia
E-mail address: david@ausvet.com.au

Vet Clin Food Anim 27 (2011) 647–654
doi:10.1016/j.cvfa.2011.07.011
0749-0720/11/$ – see front matter © 2011 Elsevier Inc. All rights reserved.

and related diseases." From a small organization of laboratory scientists, the association has grown to embrace members from over 30 countries and from diverse fields of interest, including livestock production, animal disease control, public health, and human gastroenterology (www.paratuberculosis.org). The association hosts and publishes the proceedings of its international colloquia every 2 to 3 years to update members and other interested people on developments in the knowledge, technology, and control of Johne's disease. Recent colloquia have been held in Spain, Denmark and Japan with the most recent in Minneapolis in 2009. The 11th colloquium will be held in Australia in 2012.

RESEARCH

The International Association for Paratuberculosis and its regular colloquia have stimulated collaborative discussion and research among members, many of whom have extended the knowledge on Johne's disease internationally through postgraduate study and sabbatical exchanges. Researchers in Asia, the Pacific, and the Americas are also participating in or benefiting from 2 large research programs recently initiated in the United States and in Europe.

The Johne's Disease Integrated Program (JDIP) has coordinated a large collaborative research and extension program since 2004 involving academic institutions across the United States (http://www.jdip.org). The 4 main collaborative research programs aim to:

1. Better understand Johne's disease epidemiology and the process of disease transmission.
2. Develop and implement new generations of diagnostic tests and methods for strain differentiation.
3. Improve understanding of the biology and pathogenesis of MAP.
4. Elucidate the immune response to MAP and evaluate and develop new generations of vaccines.

The European Union's Food Quality and Safety collaborative research program, ParaTB Tools, commenced in 2006 with 28 partner institutions from 16 countries and has projects covering 5 themes[9]:

1. Standardization, harmonization, and improvement of laboratory diagnosis of paratuberculosis in livestock
2. Interaction between host and pathogen in ruminants infected with MAP: development of improved diagnostic tests
3. Inactivation of MAP in milk and dairy products
4. Risk and control
5. Characterization of the interaction between humans with Crohn's disease (CD) and MAP to establish whether a causal relationship is present.

CONTROL

The desire to provide the dairy industry worldwide with up to date advice on Johne's disease and its control led the International Dairy Federation to sponsor a series of collaborative activities from 1999. The resulting proceedings outlined the then-current state of knowledge and its application to on-farm control in several countries.[10,11] In turn, the World Organization for Animal Health (OIE) then sought to improve its guidelines on population-level disease control in the chapter on paratuberculosis in the Terrestrial Animal Health Code. The existing Code chapter recommended movement certification, based on the recent known history of Johne's disease in the herd of origin, supplemented by negative tests on the animals being traded. Given the subclinical nature of Johne's disease and the low sensitivity of diagnostic tests at the individual animal level, certification based on these requirements is of limited value and may inadvertently contribute to increased spread.

The OIE subsequently considered a new Code chapter that recommended more valid herd level assessments but, 5 years ago, removed the text of the old chapter. Following another review in 2009, the OIE confirmed this position[12] so that the code chapter now only contains a reference to the terrestrial manual.[13] Inappropriate movement requirements, on one hand, do little to validly assess and manage high-risk movements of breeding animals, while, on the other hand, can impose unwarranted restrictions on low-risk movements.

While the movement standards have not been resolved, the OIE continues to provide guidance and support for diagnostic standards for Johne's disease through its *Manual of Diagnostic Tests and Vaccines for Terrestrial Animals 2010*[14] supported by, reference laboratories and experts in several countries.

Also flowing from the IDF's work ten years ago has been an informal ParaTB Forum that has been held in association with the World Dairy Congress in Shanghai in 2006 and with the International Colloquium on Paratuberculosis in 2009.[15] These forums bring together managers from countries that have implemented Johne's disease control programs to review and critique how improved knowledge and tools have been applied in their national control and assurance programs and to learn from one another's challenges and successes. As outlined below, successfully controlling Johne's disease has posed formidable challenges in several countries.

NATIONAL APPROACHES

Several countries have developed and refined national strategies to deal with Johne's disease during the past 2 decades. These have varied depending on the particular country's livestock production and trading environment and whether livestock industry and/or governments have been the major drivers. In general, government animal health services have largely led programs aimed at protecting uninfected regions (such as northern and western Australia) or at eradicating infection from populations with low prevalences of Johne's disease such as in Sweden and Japan. In other countries, such as Austria,[16] governments have recently been heavily involved in the early stages of response to rapidly increasing occurrence of disease.

In contrast, programs aimed at managing the risk of spread and contamination in endemically infected livestock populations in western Europe have been largely led by the national livestock industry organizations or, as is happening in Australia, are now becoming increasingly dependent on industry leadership and funding as government commitment changes. Food safety authorities in several developed countries have been monitoring developments related to Crohn's disease but have generally not mandated standards to manage human exposure to MAP, preferring to encourage ongoing on-farm risk management programs and good food processing practice.

National strategies generally have one or more of the following aims:

- Improving knowledge and understanding of MAP and developing tools to better manage MAP infection and contamination and its impacts
- Managing the risk of unacceptable levels of MAP occurring in food products

- Preventing and controlling the effects of Johne's disease on animal production and welfare
- Preventing and reducing the occurrence of MAP in herds and regions
- Demonstrating the low-risk status of breeding herds and flocks
- Eradicating MAP from herds and/or regional livestock populations.

In the majority of countries, programs have been directed at the dairy and beef cattle industries but significant Johne's disease programs have also been implemented for sheep (eg, in Australia), goats (Norway), deer (New Zealand) and South American camelids (Australia).

CONTROL AND RISK ASSESSMENT IN ENDEMICALLY INFECTED POPULATIONS

Johne's disease is well established in intensive cattle production systems in most countries, especially in dairy herds. The Netherlands, the United States, and Australia have been in the vanguard of controlling endemic Johne's disease, and each country's strategies have evolved substantially over time. In the United States and Australia, animal disease control is largely a constitutional responsibility of the states, rather than the federal government, and the initial steps to control Johne's disease were largely unilateral state-based regulatory programs. Interstate movement regulations were also implemented in the United States and Australia in the hope of reducing spread between regions.

A major problem for these types of regulatory programs resulted from a focus on and discrimination against herds that were officially known to be infected. Test-and-cull programs also were optimistic that MAP-infected herds could transition out of their infected status to "freedom" over several years. Regrettably, the sensitivity of tests and the cost effectiveness of programs were poor, so most owners saw little benefit in, and many downsides from, confirming MAP infection in their herds. A consequence was that most infected herds remained undetected. They were not engaged in actively controlling the infection and continued to sell infected animals.

In the mid to late 1990s the Dutch, U.S., and Australian programs took an important step towards more modern risk assessment and management of Johne's disease as a subclinical infection in endemically infected regions. For instance, within infected herds, a common recommendation to cull all test-positive cows before their next calving was refined to using the individual serologic or fecal culture results as indicators of the risk that a particular cow was a major contributor to shedding of MAP and therefore to contamination of milk and to infection of replacement calves. The focus also shifted from a focus on whether a herd was known to be MAP-infected toward probabilities that herds may be infected or that the prevalence would exceed a certain prevalence. The Australian Market Assurance Programs and the U.S. Voluntary Herd Status Program outlined how herd owners could objectively and transparently demonstrate a specified low risk of their herds being infected with MAP.[17,18]

The Dutch animal health service has taken this risk assessment a step further after a 1990s longitudinal study of test negative herds found that most of them were actually infected.[19] The Netherlands has moved to a program that classifies milk-producing herds as high risk (red herds) or low risk (green), not of being infected per se, but rather of contaminating bulk milk at a level above which pasteurization would eliminate organisms.[20] Risk assessment is also the basis of control programs in Ontario and the western provinces in Canada.[21]

In the face of a high prevalence of infection, the voluntary Danish cattle industry program has also taken a probabilistic approach to classifying herds and cows by risk, depending on antibody levels in milk.[22] Quarterly herd recording samples are tested for evidence of a range of infections including Johne's disease and the participating herds' risks published on the industry website.

Although most international attention has been paid to Johne's disease in cattle, infection with S type MAP, is endemic in major sheep-producing countries including Spain,[23] Australia,[24] New Zealand,[25] and South Africa,[5] and an Indian Bison type organism is common in sheep and goats in India.[6] Small ruminant production systems often provide few opportunities to manage individual animals and vaccination has been a more important tool to reduce the impact of disease within infected flocks and herds. From 1966, Iceland enforced a strict vaccination program in sheep, combined with movement controls that eliminated clinical disease however subsequent surveillance confirmed that the S-type infection had not been eradicated.[26]

ASSURANCE FOR DOMESTIC ANIMAL TRADE

Unlike most developed livestock-producing countries, the livestock populations over a large part of northern and western Australia have demonstrably little or no Johne's disease. To protect that status, movements are regulated into those areas so that introduced animals have only a low probability of being infected with paratuberculosis. In turn, this pressure gradient has extended southward and eastward through pedigree breeding herds and flocks, encouraging many to provide an appropriate level of assurance. To this end, the Australian Johne's Disease Market Assurance Programs commenced in 1996 to provide a transparent national standard for owner declarations based on herd and flock biosecurity and negative testing.[17] In the past 5 years, more broadly applicable and attractive herd and flock risk scoring schemes have been developed for the dairy, sheep, and goat industries.[27,28] These cover a wider range of herd statuses from herds and flocks that are infected but undertaking no control (score 0) through to high-level market assurance program herds and flocks. The "pure beef" sector (that has little or no contact with dairy cattle) and alpaca populations in Australia have very little Johne's and have developed assurance schemes based on herd biosecurity. Farmers are encouraged to use nationally agreed animal health statements to declare their assurance level when selling stock. The effectiveness of these schemes is about to be critically reviewed but suffice to say that there have been very different outcomes in different livestock sectors and in different regions.

REGIONAL DISEASE PREVENTION AND ERADICATION

Most countries have struggled to effectively control the spread of endemic Johne's disease once it has established in its livestock populations. In Australia, for instance, the sheep strain was probably introduced about 50 years ago but its known distribution remained quite localized in central New South Wales for a further 15 years. Since then, however, it has been progressively detected over a wide area of southern Australia, despite the efforts of initial regulatory programs and later voluntary industry–government programs to control it.[29] The estimated prevalence of infected flocks in large parts of New South Wales and Victoria is now over 30%.[30]

Several regions and countries have adopted energetic programs to protect their livestock populations and limit the spread of Johne's disease before it has established widely. Sweden has successfully eradicated the cattle strain that was introduced in imported cattle in the 1970s,[31] and Norway maintains a program to control Johne's disease in goats and prevent its spillover into cattle.[32] Japan commenced a national program of surveillance testing of all cattle herds every 5 years in 1997, with follow-up test and cull programs in herds identified as infected with a view to eradicating Johne's disease.[33] Northern and western Australia are officially declared protected and free zones for the cattle strain of MAP, and these regions have successfully prevented the establishment of infection by movement controls and stamping out infection when detected. Queensland and South Australia have taken similar action to protect their sheep flocks from ovine infection.

SUMMARY

The epidemiology and pathogenesis of Johne's disease facilitated its spread with livestock movements across the globe during the twentieth century, initially from Europe and subsequently from other developed livestock exporting countries. In the past 20 years, international collaboration in research and disease control methods has increased. The previous international guidelines on movement certification for Johne's disease have been removed from the OIE Terrestrial Animal Health Code but are yet to be replaced by standards that will effectively contribute to reducing the risk of international spread. Over the past 2 decades, individual countries have conducted a range of programs aimed at controlling the spread of Johne's disease between herds and flocks, with the more successful being those that have energetically addressed the disease before it has established. In endemically infected regions, control of the disease within infected herds and flocks focuses on reducing the impacts on animal welfare and productivity and in reducing contamination of the farm environment and of farm products. This is undertaken through reducing the exposure of young animals, vaccination, and/or identifying and removing animals that are most likely contributing to heavy contamination of the farm and environment. Collaboration among the international community of researchers, government regulators, and livestock industry leaders has significantly contributed to improved understanding of Johne's disease and to more innovative strategies to deal with it.

ACKNOWLEDGMENTS

The author wishes to thank Animal Health Australia for supporting this paper and many colleagues around the world who, over the years, have generously shared their experience and insights on controlling Johne's disease.

REFERENCES

1. Available at: http://www.oie.int/wahis/public.php?page_disease_status_lists. Accessed November 24, 2010.
2. Albiston HE. Johne's disease. In: Diseases of domestic animals in Australia, Part 5, Vol 1, bacterial diseases. Canberra: Commonwealth Department of Health; 1965. p. 150–62.
3. Kennedy DJ, Benedictus G. Control of *Mycobacterium avium* subsp. *paratuberculosis* infection in agricultural species. Rev Sci Tech Off Int Epiz 2001;20:151–79.
4. Shahmoradi AH, Arefpajohi R, Tadayon K, et al. Paratuberculosis in Holstein-Friesian cattle farms in Central Iran. Trop Anim Health Prod 2008;40:169–73.
5. Michel AL, Bastianello SS. Paratuberculosis in sheep: an emerging disease in South Africa. Vet Microbiol 2000;77:299–307.
6. Singh AV, Singh SV, Singh PK et al. Genotype diversity in Indian isolates of *Mycobacterium avium* subspecies *paratuberculosis* recovered from domestic and wild ruminants from different agro-climatic regions. Comp Immunol Microbiol Infect Dis 2010; Sep 8. [Epub ahead of print].

7. Lee KW, Jung BY. Seroprevalence of *Mycobacterium avium* subspecies *paratuberculosis* in cattle in Korea. Vet Rec 2009;165:661–2.
8. Chiodini RJ. Crohn's disease and the mycobacterioses: a review and comparison of two disease entities. Clin Microbiol Rev 1989; 2:90–117.
9. Available at: http://www.vigilanciasanitaria.es/paratbtool. Accessed November 18, 2010.
10. International Dairy Federation. *Mycobacterium paratuberculosis*. Bulletin 362/2001. Brussels: Author; 2001.
11. International Dairy Federation. On farm control and diagnosis of paratuberculosis. Bulletin 364/2001. Brussels: Author; 2001.
12. Available at: http://www.oie.int/downld/SC/2009/A_TAHSC_Sept%202009_Introduction.pdf. Accessed November 24, 2010.
13. Available at: http://www.oie.int/eng/normes/mcode/en_chapitre_1.8.9.htm. Accessed November 18, 2010.
14. Available at: http://www.oie.int/eng/normes/mmanual/2008/pdf/2.01.11_PARATB.pdf. Accessed November 18, 2010.
15. International Dairy Federation. Monitoring success of paratuberculosis programs. Proceedings of the Second ParaTB Forum, Minneapolis, August 2009. Nielsen SS, editor. Bulletin 441/2009. Brussels: Author; 2009.
16. Khol JL, Damoser J, Dünser M, et al. Paratuberculosis, a notifiable disease in Austria--current status, compulsory measures and first experiences. Prev Vet Med 2007;82:302–7.
17. Kennedy DJ, Neumann GB. The Australian National Johne's Disease Market Assurance Program. In: Proceedings 5th International Colloquium on Paratuberculosis. Melbourne: 1999. p. 121-31.
18. Kovich DA, Wells SJ, Friendshuh K. Evaluation of the Voluntary Johne's Disease Herd Status Program as a source of replacement cattle. J Dairy Sci 2006;89:3466–70.
19. Kalis CH, Collins MT, Barkema HW, et al. Certification of herds as free of *Mycobacterium paratuberculosis* infection: actual pooled faecal results versus certification model predictions. Prev Vet Med 2004;65:189–204.
20. Weber MF, Nielen M, Velthuis AG, et al. Milk quality assurance for paratuberculosis: simulation of within-herd infection dynamics and economics. Vet Res 2008;39:12. Epub 2008 Jan 29.
21. Sorge US, Mount J, Kelton DF, et al.Veterinarians' perspective on a voluntary Johne's disease prevention program in Ontario and western Canada. Can Vet J 2010;51:403–5.
22. Kudahl AB, Nielsen SS, Østergaard SJ. Economy, efficacy, and feasibility of a risk-based control program against paratuberculosis. J Dairy Sci 2008;91:4599–609.
23. Sevilla I, Singh SV, Garrido JM, et al. Molecular typing of Mycobacterium avium subspecies paratuberculosis strains from different hosts and regions. Rev Sci Tech 2005;24:1061–6.
24. Cousins DV, Williams SN, Hope A, et al. DNA fingerprinting of Australian isolates of Mycobcaterium avium subsp. paratuberculosis using IS900 RFLP. Aust Vet J 2000;78:184–90.
25. de Lisle GWN. Johne's disease in New Zealand: the past, present and a glimpse into the future. N Z Vet J 2002;50(3 Suppl):53–6.
26. Gunnarsson E, Fridriksdóttir V, Sigurdarson S. Control of paratuberculosis in Iceland Acta Vet Scand 2003;44:255.

27. Kennedy D, Citer L. Paratuberculosis control measures in Australia. In: Behr MA, Collins DM, editors. Paratuberculosis:organism, disease, control. Wallingford: CAB International; 2009. p. 330–43.

28. Available at: http://www.animalhealthaustralia.com.au/programs/jd/jd_home.cfm. Accessed November 18, 2010.

29. Sergeant ES. Ovine Johne's disease in Australia: the first 20 years. Aust Vet J 2001;79;484–91.

30. Available at: http://www.animalhealthaustralia.com.au/programs/jd/naojd/ojd_prevalence.cfm. Accessed November 24, 2010.

31. Sternberg S, Viske D. Control strategies for paratuberculosis in Sweden. Acta Vet Scand 2003;44:247–9.

32. Tharaldsen J, Djønne B, Fredriksen B, et al. The National Paratuberculosis Program in Norway. Acta Vet Scand 2003;44:243–6.

33. Kobayashi S, Tsutsui T, Yamamoto A, et al. Epidemiologic indicators associated with within-farm spread of Johne's disease in dairy farms in Japan. J Vet Med Sci 2007;69:1255–8.

Index

Note: Page numbers of article titles are in **boldface** type.

Vet Clin Food Anim 27 (2011) 655–663
doi:10.1016/S0749-0720(11)00053-3
0749-0720/11/$ – see front matter © 2011 Elsevier Inc. All rights reserved.

vetfood.theclinics.com

Printed and bound by CPI Group (UK) Ltd, Croydon, CR0 4YY

03/10/2024

01040455-0013